When Life Hands You Lemons...

...and other trite bullshit we tell ourselves to get through cancer.

Katie Weber

Kila Springs

Kila Springs Press is an imprint of the Kila Springs Group,
Placerville, CA.
E-mail: press@kilasprings.net

Cover: Lauren Ruebe

First Edition

ISBN 978-1-7338479-2-6
Library of Congress Control Number: 2019948934

For Will, my love, my rock, my life.

Acknowledgements

First and foremost, I want to acknowledge my immediate community of family and friends who are and have been a pillar of strength and support my whole life, but especially during my health crises. A silver lining of battling a disease like this is that your team comes out in droves and I am blessed with an all-star team. Always have been.

Of that team, I have to give special acknowledgement to my husband, Will, who is THE best man to walk this earth. Sorry, but I won't budge on it. Will, you and I struggle through this together and it is the hardest times, but you have never wavered. Not in 2011 after just three years together and not again in 2016 when we had just decided to make it forever official. The fact that you never flinched is why I am able to fight and go on like a fucking badass every day.

And of course, my mom, dad and brother who are the most supportive family I could have asked for and in whose relationships I've grown through this process. My parents inspired in me a love of reading and writing that has endured through time. Thank you.

I thank everyone who believed in me and helped make this dream a reality including my good friends, Brian Henderson and Kyra Mirante, for editing my things (you can blame them and cancer for any typos), my old friend, Lauren Ruebe, for designing the cover with me, and my uncle, David Ollier Weber, for publishing my book through his Kila Springs Press.

I also want to thank a new(er) friend, Randi Eseltine, for helping me market this book and figure out how to brag about myself (just a little bit).

Finally, I want to acknowledge and thank the writer Roxanne Gay. Her style, critical reflections and voice were/are incredibly inspiring to me in this process. Especially her collection of essays *Bad Feminist*, whose structure I borrowed from throughout much of this book. Like all my favorite authors, she has been able to translate the human experience into language and stories that others can identify with.

I. INTRODUCTION

"It is what it is."

Perspective

I think it's important for me to say that I write this book from one perspective: mine.

I know that's what memoirs are, but it feels important to acknowledge that, with a disease like cancer, there is no universal truth. Every type of cancer is different. Every person. Every experience. I've just learned a hell of a lot going through all of this and if anything good can come out of it, it's awareness, perspective, and knowledge. So, I guess I feel a bit of a responsibility to write it all down.

Plus, about 5 percent of cancer diagnoses in this country are in young people ages 15-39 (https://www.cancer.gov/types/aya), and yet, the writings (or so I've found) for young adults are scant or non-existent. It's hard to find anything that "real talks" this situation and understands how the experience for someone young—especially someone in their 20's—is different than a "typical" cancer experience. Sure, there are some common things that seem universal to cancer like chemo and radiation and ports and hospitals, but even those things are not necessarily universal. And I think the way cancer affects your life and psychology is just different when you are a young adult. Again, my opinions, my perspective.

My story very much defines my twenties and when I tell you a little bit more about it, you'll see why.

When I was 23, I was having some weird, disconcerting symptoms, so I went to the E.R. at Swedish Hospital and was almost immediately rushed to the neuro-ICU to deal with a large (kiwi-sized!) mass on my cerebellum. Which, for those of you who don't know, is the back of your brain, lower down near your neck, that controls certain motor skills and balance. And lots of other things I'm finding.

I could not be rushed into surgery because fluid had built up in my brain, causing lots of swelling and they had to drain it before surgery was possible. The time between the emergency room and waking up from surgery is very vague, because I was almost completely out of it. At one point I was asked what year it was and I said, with full conviction and certainty, 2003. It was 2011. I barely remember this moment.

What I HAVE gathered is that I was not myself and all my family and friends were incredibly concerned about me. There was the risk that I would come out of surgery a different person. There was risk that the "mass" was cancerous. (Surprise, surprise, it was!) There was a lot of fear to go around and I know people I love (and who, I'm grateful to say, love me) really feel that. It will always be something I wish I could undo.

My official diagnosis: desmoplastic medulloblastoma in the cerebellum. It's a tumor that occurs most commonly among children, but even then, I was told by an expert at Seattle Children's Hospital (Dr. Sarah Leary), there are only about 400 cases of medulloblastoma per year in the U.S. across all age groups. So, it's like being 1 in a million for all of the wrong reasons.

After surgery, I had some time to recover. Then I went into, I believe, 33 days of radiation.

Radiation therapy is terrible in terms of how it makes you feel. An MRI is as close as you get to the experience, but still is not the same. After radiation you're tired, you have a headache, and you DEFINITELY don't feel like yourself. I was not on the most modern anti-nausea medication, so I spent the whole first night throwing up.

For me, radiation had a smell. The people who worked there said they did not smell it, but I think it was kind of like getting used to our own B.O., because I remember smelling that smell before I even got into the office, and it made me feel sick every time.

After radiation, I did three months of intense chemotherapy. I slept a lot, and I watched the entirety of *Friday Night Lights* in just a couple of weeks. Clear eyes, full hearts, fuck cancer. (This is a *Friday Night Lights*—the show, not the movie—reference. If you have not seen the show, do yourself a favor, and watch it. It is SO good. Also, my writing is riddled with pop culture references. If you get them, great. If you don't but want to, I suggest Google.)

After chemotherapy, I had another MRI and voila! Cancer free. It felt amazing to hear that. But there's always a chance of a return and one must be ready for anything.

This is where the follow-up begins. And it's not terrible, but it's no one's favorite. For three years I had an MRI every three months, to keep an eye on me. Every time, the scan was perfect. After three years, I dropped down to every six months. After five years, it would go to every year; hit 10 and they stop scanning you at all.

I was certain I would beat the odds. I mean, come on! I was young, athletic, a *vegetarian* (mostly), and I avoided sugar. I was like the "yahh, no thanks, cancer" poster child.

In July of 2016, I had my 4.5-year scan. I was feeling good: engaged to be married and active—I rode my bike to the hospital! I always had good scans. I mean, scans were always scary, but after nearly five years of nothing, they had become routine and I'd had time to get used to who I was and what my life would be in Seattle. My hair had grown back, I biked a lot, and I finally felt like I knew what I wanted to do with my life, career-wise. But at this 4.5-year scan they saw something that wasn't perfect. When they scanned me two months later, it had slightly grown.

The docs didn't like it. It *could* be scar tissue, but it could also not be. Unfortunately, the only real way to know is to go in and check it out. Unfortunately, when cancer is in your brain, "checking it out" means brain surgery. As you can imagine, that is no small thing.

We did it. A biopsy. And what no one thought was cancer was indeed cancer. This was in December of 2016. There I was, at age 29 this time, back with cancer.

This time around has been very different from when I was 23. No emergency surgeries. More decisions. More changes to my life. This second time around has also given me more time to learn about and ponder the oddities of this life. And the pain. And the struggle.

Cancer has taken more from me the second time around, and everything is less emergent. When I was 23-years-young and zipping through it, I lost very little and didn't have the time—or maturity—to think about what cancer really means in this world. Don't get me wrong, I do not want to be defined by cancer, but I would be lying if I said that it hasn't affected my psychology or my life in any real way.

Right now, the treatment process is long and uncertain. I did some chemotherapy regimens that may have worked, may have not. The world of cancer is a world of uncertainty and surrender of control. I am weak and often feel really tired, but otherwise, you would likely think I was fine.

In this journey to understand myself and this life I'm forced to live, I've learned a lot. I hope you can, too. And I hope this book provides a modicum of a resource for young adults who get cancer and feel totally alone in a world of new job opportunities, partying and dancing all night, endless energy, and the changes and hopes that bring young people to adventurous places. I had and have great friends, an amazing partner and a supportive family. But I know I still felt like someone apart. And probably always will.

II. CELLULAR DATA

"The Devil is in the details."

A medical dictionary

After so much time frequenting hospitals, it's easy for me to forget that most people haven't spent as much time with doctors as I have. I tend to use medical terms casually, because I think people just know them. The sad reality is that I now know a hell of a lot more about hospitals and treatments than the general population, including my friends. That's good for them.

I am always happy to clarify something, for anyone. But it's also good to actually understand what someone you care about is saying, so I thought a little "glossary" of a sort would be useful. This isn't only to understand cancer vocabulary, but also to be able to follow what's going on in this book. The list is not exhaustive. And, by the way, this is all just from what I know. I am in no way a scientist, doctor, or expert. Also not sure I want to be. But thank you, all you people who are.

Medulloblastoma: This is the type of brain cancer I have. As mentioned in the intro, it is typically a child's cancer and is very rare among adults. Which means there's not a ton of research out there about treating it in adults. Good stuff.

My medulloblastoma is technically "desmoplastic medulloblastoma" which I have truly never understood. I don't do a lot of internet research on my own tumor (you can imagine why), so this one is up to you if "desmoplastic" makes a huge difference to your understanding.

Cerebellum: The cerebellum is at the base of the skull, right near the spinal cord. This part of your brain is mostly responsible for fine motor skills and balance, though it also controls other things, too.

Basic brain anatomy has never been my strength. Also, human brains are crazy, amazing places.

My cancer was found in the cerebellum, which means I have now had brain surgery in that region twice. Currently, my left hand is shaky (because the cerebellum controls our motor function) which might be forever or might be temporary. Same with my balance. My (phenomenal) typing speed has decreased from 100 wpm to 40 wpm. This incenses me, though there are certainly other, more important things in life.

Ataxia: I have this right now (August 2019). It is its own disease that often comes after a stroke, but can just happen… 'cause why not? It is very common with brain cancer, and involves a great loss of coordination and balance. The best way I can describe it is that it's like putting your forehead to a wiffle ball bat, spinning around a bunch of times, getting dizzy and trying to run in a straight line. The only difference is that, in that situation, you know that you are dizzy. With ataxia, you often think your balance is fine.

MRI (Magnetic Resonance Imaging): A process by which doctors scan your body using some insane, NASA-discovered* technology to see very detailed pictures of what's going on beneath all of that skin and bone. The machines are very large and very loud with smallish tube-shaped openings that a technician helps you get into. You lie on a bed/cot-like surface and you are remotely pushed in and out of the tube. It's a trip and not a favorite of the claustrophobic (me! hehe).

# of times I've had an MRI: At least 40 times that I can count, but probably more.

---

*I have no idea if NASA or any of their research was actually involved in the invention of the MRI. That's me just spouting.**

That will happen a lot, so do not take these "facts" to be Facts. I will double check and cite where I can, but this isn't a research paper. Sorry!*

***[Editor's note: MRI was not invented by NASA.]

My MRI Story

I know the drill. I typically schedule my scans for early Sunday morning because a) I don't have to take work off, which is especially helpful when the scans are hours long (which they are when I have to have my spine AND my brain scanned) and b) I'm sleepy on Sunday mornings, so I'm more likely to sleep through some of the scan.

When I walk into the MRI department, they always ask me to fill out the same form, with the same questions about history of disease and how much metal I've decided to pierce through my skin. The form is always green. I wonder if they ever run out of that green paper and have to print it on white?

I've only ever had one technician in the history of technicians who remembered who I was and knew that I had done this about a million times (clearly an exaggeration considering I just told you it's in the 40s). He was from Louisiana (Baton Rouge, I believe) and his voice was very kind and comforting. He had a daughter in her teen years. I think he imagined her in my place when I was lying on the MRI bed. I wonder what happened to him.

Now I get techs who feel the need to explain every bit of the process to me. Which, on an intellectual level, I understand, they're just doing their job. On an emotional level, I find these people so annoying.

Yes, I know, my nose ring is metal, but it's hard to get out and it's never been an issue. My cartilage earring, too? Yeah, I know it will create a refraction on the scan, but it has never been a problem — in the 5+ years I've been doing this. Promise, we're good.

I mean, I come freakin' DRESSED for the occasion so I don't have to put on hospital robes. Sports bra, leggings, t-shirt – no metal! I know the drill! One time a tech put my bra up next to the machine and I observed the powerful pull of its underwire. That was creepy. I would not want to lie to you about my underwire.

The techs always eventually relent to me, realizing that I've done this too many times and I'm fed up. I just want to get it over with. They're always nice people, just doing what they're supposed to do, and my annoyance is always misplaced. I'm sorry, tech people. It's not you. It's the cancer. I wonder how many times they've heard THAT one??

I get up onto the little metal table that I'm going to lie on for the next 40 minutes to three hours, depending on the scan. They've already taken my glasses by then, so I'm just going on feel (since I'm basically blind – a malformity the MRI machine can't detect!). The table and room are always freezing and I'm always just shivering, waiting for a blanket or sheet.

They try to make me as comfortable as possible, with a cushion under my knees and padding wherever I ask for it, but it's not that easy to be comfortable, lying on your back, in a plastic mask they have fitted to my head (to keep my head still), an IV in my arm (for a contrast injection), earplugs in, and foam blocks between my ears and the plastic cage to keep my head in the juuust right position (I usually end up with about an inch total of wiggle room from left to right). It's uncomfortable, but I guess I'm used to it by now. Kind of feels like a safe space. Oddly.

Before I start the scans, I get that IV set up, as mentioned. Contrast is a dye they put in your bloodstream to help differentiate between normal/healthy tissue and abnormal tissue. I don't really understand it, but I know it exists and that they use it every time I get a scan.

Cold alcohol swab. Quick stick. IV in. Saline rinse, to be sure it's flowing properly. One of the strangest things about this process is that you can taste and smell things as they are injected into your bloodstream. With the saline, I taste and smell salt every time. The contrast tastes and smells more like something metallic. Like maybe if you sucked on iron tablets or something. I don't do that, so I'm not sure.

The scans themselves are noisy and close-quartered. It's my brain they're getting pictures of so I'm pushed all the way into the tube. I'm like a human burrito! Which is a fun way to think about it, since I can't move my head or really anything else. I actually don't mind it in there, which is a true act of zen for me, because I have a pretty decent case of claustrophobia. The first few times I got a long scan, I took some Ativan to help me chill out, but now, I just close my eyes, remind myself the position is temporary and I can always escape it, and try to sleep.

Some people find the MRI machine's noises really loud and annoying, but I've come to treat them like my own personal form of music. Those people are not wrong. The machine is very loud and its machine noises are very annoying. They are kind of a non-melodic mix of RJD2, Girl Talk, and Skrillex, but the beat never drops. (I recognize those are all very out-of-date music references, but I'm kind of out of date). One thing I appreciate about them is that they are very monotonous, so I can treat it kind of like an odd noise machine. And fall asleep.

My last scan, I fell asleep for about an hour, but it was an estimated 3-4 hour scan. So, I woke up and started to recognize how uncomfortable my body was. Odd pressure points on my bones, itches all over that I couldn't scratch, and a very dry, thirsty mouth/throat.

I decided to press the little button that tells the tech "I need out!" I wasn't bailing on the scan, not after all of that, but I did need a little break. He afforded me that, but wouldn't allow me to take my mask/cage off to move my head. So, in one of the more dehumanizing experiences I've had in an MRI room, this technician (NOT a nurse), fed me water from a straw through my mask-cage. My mouth was grasping at the straw, telling him I needed it close as water sort of dribbled down my chin. I felt like a toddler. Or a dying 90-year-old. Either way, it wasn't the best. But is anything the best about cancer?

Heated blankets. Those are the best.

So, I go back inside the machine to finish the scan. For the next hour I try to rest, mostly just count free-throws (or whatever comes to me) and make up words to go along with the monotonous songs of the machine.

Poor machine. It does so much to help us and we all hate it. I hear your song, MRI machine, and it is (not) beautiful.

When I'm finished, I have very little to show for it other than some lower back pain and a desire to scratch every surface of my body and dance around a little bit. Results from the scan don't come until I see the doctor.

So I wait.

LP (Lumbar puncture): Most people would probably just call this a spinal tap. They are very scary and the needle is pretty long, but they are not AS bad as they are rumored to be. Unfortunately, their relative badness is often dependent on who is doing it. I say "unfortunately," because we often have no control over who does it. One time, I had an LP I didn't even notice. Another time, I had one that was really painful and I twitched a lot. So, who really knows? I would suggest a light sedative, either way.

Hydrocephalus: In layman's terms, this means just what it sounds like: water on the brain. This can happen any time the ventricles in your brain get blocked up from something like cancer cells, but it can also not be that, and so they drain the excess fluid that builds up in your brain. A normal body does this on its own. MY brain is extra special and requires a *shunt* (def. below) to properly do this. Symptoms of hydrocephalus include confusion, difficulty committing things to short-term memory, and severe weakness. All things I deal with daily, regardless!

Shunt: Merriam-Webster defines a shunt as "a surgical passage created to divert a bodily fluid (such as blood) from one vessel or part to another" (Merriam-Webster's website—I wonder if they enjoy that accidental pun as much as I... probably not) and that definition seems as good to me as anything I might come up with. In my case, it is water/excess fluid, not blood, and that fluid is diverted through tubes to my stomach cavity. I don't understand a lot about it except that it was the most painful surgery I've ever had (and I've replaced my ACL).

Contrast Dye: As described in my MRI story, this is a dye injected intravenously to help make the image easier to read, which makes the disease easier to find. There are a lot more scientific things about the way contrast works that you are welcome to research.

I get this dye every time I get an MRI. It's not a big deal. Though I imagine it is for people who are allergic to it.

Radiologist: The person licensed to read your medical imaging and write up a summary for the oncologist and for the patient. Radiologists also read x-rays and probably other things.

This person reads every one of my MRIs, but I am only allowed to know the results at a doctor's appointment, because the techs, who take my exam in the moment, do not necessarily have an M.D. and it might be a little bit before the radiologist looks at my scan.

Oncologist: This is my main man (in my case, he's a man). He's the cancer doc who is sort of running the show. Typically, oncologists are mainly in charge of chemo treatment and the overall "how you doing?" aspect of seeing a doctor once/month.

Mine is named Dr. Graber, at UW Hospital, and he's a good doctor and a very good man.

Radiation Oncologist: This is a whole 'nother doctor involved in treatment, but usually just at the very beginning. If radiation is part of the treatment plan (almost always is with brain tumors), the radiation oncologist figures all of those details out—how long, how strong, etc. They also give tattoo dots on the torso to make sure the patient is lined up properly every time. I've never been more amused in a hospital than when a nurse in scrubs and rubber gloves had to break out the tattoo gun and tat me up in the middle of the room.

I've had the same Radiation Oncologist twice, Dr. Landis at Swedish Medical Center, and he's amazing. My mom has a crush on him. Can't blame her!

Port (port-a-cath): Not all cancer patients get a port, but if extensive chemotherapy is part of the treatment plan, then they'll probably get one or at least have discussed it. A port is a catheter—a long tube—connected to a reservoir. Mine is kind of shaped like a metal Rolo*, though I'm sure they come in all different shapes. This tube is surgically connected to your aorta (or other strong bloodline) and the little Rolo sits just under the skin in your upper chest, nearish to your collarbone. It is much easier to "access" the port than to find a new vein every time for treatment or any time blood is given (or taken). One time at chemo, before I had my second port, they poked

---

Editor's note: A small chocolate/caramel candy shaped like a blunt cone.

me FIVE times trying to find a vein that worked well enough to administer the drug.

I had a port in 2011 and I have a new one now. When they took the old one out in '12, I got a tattoo right over the scar. They were nice enough this time to not cut over my tattoo.

Grand-Mal Seizure: A physically visible seizure that is probably exactly what you think of when you think of a seizure. Can include: spasming, locked jaw or face, strange and sort of frozen hand tics, and general "out of it"-ness.

Subclinical Seizure: The kind of seizure that happens in your brain but is not visible to anyone, sometimes not even the person who is having the seizure. I, personally, could recognize my subclinical seizures, but according to my epileptologist, that is rare.

I have had both of these things. Only one grand-mal seizure which was so, so scary for me AND my husband. I've had lots of subclinical seizures while in the hospital, apparently.

Bell's Palsy/Facial Palsy: This doesn't actually have anything to do with cancer, particularly, but I think it's fairly common with brain cancer since our brain controls so many nerves and such. I'm not actually sure what's going on with me, but whatever it is I basically cannot fully move my face. So… no smiling, no crying, tough to chew. I look like an AI Bot who had its circuits short out. Bell's Palsy usually cures itself within six months, but I'm headed into YEAR THREE, so maybe it's not actually Bell's Palsy. Maybe it's that my nerves are so mad at me!!

Epileptologist: This is just what it sounds like—a neurologist who specializes in epilepsy and other neurological disorders that cause seizures. Makes sense, though I had no idea it was even a word.

My doctor is monitoring the anti-seizure medicine, which is something I'm not sure I need to be on. That's not a conversation for this time, but this happens when you have lots of medical issues coming at ya—sometimes there are just meds you can't deny. Luckily, we are on the path to reducing my dose in hopes of eventually getting off of it all together.

Immunocompromised: This happens when a patient's white blood cell count (the germ fighters) gets too low. This happens a lot to cancer patients, because chemotherapies often cause the good guys to die along with the bad. If this happens too much, one is "immunocompromised" in that it is much easier for that person to get sick or acquire an infection. That's why you may see a lot of cancer patients with masks on in public. Or not see them at all, because they are hiding from our germy, germy world.

I have been immunocompromised only once (maybe twice). Never wore a mask in public, because I wasn't ordered to and I'm stubborn anyway.

That's all for now. There is all SORTS of insurance jargon/hospitalese that I know I've learned by now, but this is not a dictionary of terrible things. It's just a short guide to my book nonsense. Feel free to Google anything confusing or new. I bet Google actually knows a lot more than I do. And I'm okay with that.

Opioids and Mental illness

Gimme that dilaudid!

I cannot say I understand addiction, because that is certainly not true. But that feeling of escape that seems to be behind many addictions I do understand. Sometimes you just want to be anywhere but where you are.

For me, in the hospital, the best way to escape from the physical and emotional pain I was in was dilaudid, which is an opioid and pain killer I only ever took under licensed supervision. You know when an opioid is kicking in because your entire body relaxes and you get kinda warm. And sleepy. It is an unreal feeling that is hard to explain to someone who has not ever experienced it. It's a very nice feeling and very powerful.

I've never been one to mess with hard drugs—I've never done anything harder than pot and after one bad experience with Vicodin, I did my entire ACL repair recovery on ibuprofen. I had decided that hard drugs do not have the same effect on me as they seem to on others. So the fact that I not only LOVE Dilaudid, but ask for it by name, shows you the power of opioids, especially when a situation sucks. This could be cancer, a less-than-ideal marriage, a thankless job, or a bad upbringing/life, in general.

People really want to blame America's opioid crisis on the medical system. And I do think that some bad doctors are to blame for over-prescription and lack of support. More than that, I think it's because we are sick as a nation. We kill ourselves in our careers, we expect ourselves to be fabulous at everything we do, and we don't spend enough time appreciating our friends, family, and community. We are racist, homophobic, misogynist, and xenophobic. How else would we react? We want to escape this ugly reality that is life.

Through cancer, I have seen that drugs are really helpful, but they are just a band aid. They don't take cancer away, they just make you forget that you have it. Same with the opioid crisis: opioids don't fix our country's problems, they just help us stop thinking about them.

In order to truly fix the opioid crisis, I believe, we need to look within. What's wrong with us that this is such a necessity? What's going on in society? What are we trying to escape?

Don't mess with steroids, ya'll

Ever heard of steroid-induced psychosis? Neither had I! But now I know allll about it.

First, I started on a steroid after radiation treatment to help with the nausea and headaches that I was having afterwards. This is typical. What's also typical is that when you are on a steroid, you slowly taper off, because, like any powerful drug that is basically giving your body a surge of dopamine/adrenaline to deal with symptoms, going cold turkey is just PAINFUL. So, you are slowly weaned from it for ~30 days.

Things that suck about steroids: You have acne like you haven't had in a while. You want to eat every salty, sugary, bad-for-you thing in your path at every moment. Your face is swollen and your eyes suddenly look very small. You're like an awkward 15-year-old who hasn't quite grown into their body. Oh and you have terrible insomnia. So you don't sleep.

BUT, what's great about steroids, is that, despite all of this, you have NO SELF DOUBT. That little voice that runs in (most of) our heads that tells you "no you shouldn't" or "nah, you can't" just kind of shuts up. I was operating as Katie at 11.* You're you, only better. Like Sammy Sosa is/was a great hitter, naturally. He just did things like take steroids and cork his bat because of the insane pressure he felt from the MLB and everyone. That's too bad. But I also get it. Steroids helped his muscles perform at 11. Honestly, I realized a lot of things about how much of what's been holding me back over the years has just been me and my own anxiety.

Because I ended up with too much steroid in my system (due to a long taper + a large, standard dose of steroids that comes with

---

Not age 11—"11" as in amped up, a notch higher than the highest level (10).

chemo, I had a psychotic break, or in medical terms, steroid-induced psychosis. Like a bad trip, I was completely detached from reality. I was saying CRAZY things about being the second coming of Christ and that only I could save the world. Yikes.

Luckily, my amazing partner and now husband, Wilson Bull, is smart and resourceful and wonderful and by turning to friends he was certain knew more about bad trips than he did (thanks K. and B.), he was able to bring me back to reality.

Just as we thought we were healing and getting love from our community (thanks Bryan, Geoff, Katie M.), my brain had had ENOUGH of all of this bullshit. I had a seizure. I remember the first one but I don't know how many I had between my apartment and the hospital. I do know EMTs entered my apartment and I was carried out on a stretcher. And then I spent 5 days in a hospital bed while they tried to figure out what was going on in my brain.

Honestly, it was a shitty situation. (A "shituation", if you will. You don't have to.) But I learned a lot going through it. I gained insight into how drug addicts feel and why it's so difficult to get off of something that makes you feel so awesome. I gained insight into people who are bi-polar and what their manic episodes must feel like. I already know what deep depression feels like. I'm good on that for now. I also, honest to Gaia, had a bit of a spiritual awakening. Which actually has nothing to do with Jesus and everything to do with love and energy and the earthly elements. (I'll tell you allll about it later.)

I'm not saying it was worth it. Fuck, it was terrible. Maybe the worst week of my life. But if I had to go through it, I might as well learn something from it. I have the heart of a teacher/life-long learner, after all. I can't help myself.

Psychosis: A story (and, also, that time I had a seizure)

It was a scary time. I don't remember much.

I'm lying in bed, feeling closer to reality. With much urgency, I say "No, Will, I'm back now, I swear, I'm back."

How many times has he heard me say that in the last 24 hours?

I'm coloring in my adult coloring book, which is good for stress. I suppose I am stressed but I really just feel far away. The signs were there. My intense focus on organizing my pens. My sudden inability to say any words. I guess the first sign wasn't all that strange, but the second was certainly not typical. The next thing I remember, my body is seizing. I can feel and see my hand making strange movements and my head locking in a position I don't want it to be in. I don't feel how hard I have clenched my jaw or bitten down on my tongue, but I sure notice how much my tongue hurts the next morning and I believe Will when he says he tried to open my mouth, but couldn't.

The EMTs arrive. They barge into my apartment like they're supposed to be there. I guess they are, but I only see strangers with a strange bed on wheels. By now, my seizure has stopped. They bring me downstairs and outside to a cold, wet night. The rain on my skin reminds me of where I live and the chill gives me goosebumps that still don't seem to have retreated completely.

One EMT forgot to bring a wheelchair, so instead I walk to the ambulance. I walk, in socks, on a wet sidewalk. I remember this, but with a reminder. The EMT is in trouble, but I am all about being a gracious patient, never complain, it's not a problem! I love walking! In retrospect, my walking to an ambulance on wet pavement in socks is inappropriate. In the moment, I am both fine and not fine. I feel closer to reality, but I know I am not entirely there.

The ambulance ride isn't long, but it's long enough for me to make a call. I call my dad. Looking back, he sounds scared and sad, but he keeps his cool.

"Dad?"

"Yes?"

"Do you remember some of my best basketball games?"

"Well, of course I do."

"Okay, can you tell me my stats from some of the best games that you remember?"

He begins. Listing off games where I had double and triple doubles. Games he remembers where I had a spectacular block or played incredible defense. Through tears, I say "I WAS pretty good, huh? Like, I was a good player."

"Of course you were! Of course."

I can hear his strained voice through the phone, wondering why I'm asking these questions and what is going on with his daughter. Retrospectively, I recognize why I needed this information. Anything to ground me in reality. Anything that seems true and normal. Stats don't lie. My dad's undying belief in me as a person and an athlete doesn't lie. I needed truth, and love, and grounding. I found that in the answers to those questions.

I wake up in a hospital bed. There are many doctors and nurses all around me. No one I recognize. This is a new medical team. For a new medical issue. I've had swelling in my brain, a kiwi-sized tumor, cancer, and lots of other reasons to visit doctors or the hospital, but I've never experienced steroid-induced psychosis or had a seizure until now.

Everyone is nice. I perceive a chill. I request another warm blanket—the only good thing about the hospital. Well, that and room service.

Time has stopped. Will is here. My mom has arrived. Should I be at work? Has someone called them? I should probably continue sleeping. My eyelids fall. I disappear into dreamless sleep. It feels cozy there. Safe. I go to a world where I don't have cancer. Where I've never had a seizure. Sleep is a kind place. A place to rest and forget and heal.

Eventually I am awoken by a technician. He explains that he will attach me to an EEG. Soreness at various spots on my head as he marks "x's" on my skull. A strange cold and uncomfortable feeling as the glue goes on. Then the spider-like attachments. Green waves begin to travel across the screen, signaling functionality. We'll call that a success.

Everyone is talking to me in a very specific way, that I can perceive, but find helpful. I don't like it, knowing I'm being handled with kid gloves, but I also recognize that they are helping me emerge from my psychosis. Helping me return to reality. Helping me get better.

I no longer have any visible seizures, not to the naked eye. No more twitching or convulsing. Instead I start to exhibit more subtle symptoms, like tapping my feet a lot, or not being able to speak momentarily, or an intense focus on repeated tasks. These moments were connected to subclinical seizures, tracked on my EEG. Over time, I could tell when these seizures were coming on. And I started to be able to control the behaviors associated with them: I notice my feet bobbing up and down, I bring them to rest. I feel I cannot speak, but I know I can, so I speak.

In my opinion, each subclinical seizure was part of the healing process. I needed it to help me control those symptoms or understand what was happening in my brain. This is just my opinion, backed by no degrees other than a B.A. and M.Ed. Oh and my own personal knowledge of how my body feels/works that no one else can ever understand actually.

I was given a clicker, to press a button whenever I felt I was having a subclinical seizure. Every click of the button, however confusing to the people in the room who could not perceive anything happening to me, corresponded with a subclinical seizure, tracked on the screen. I've been told this is not common. It is surprising. It always feels great to excel at things!

I need to be put on a different anti-seizure medication. The one they put me on is working, but it's not good for long-term use. Try another.

Instant intense ringing in my ears. My vision is blurred, like I'm crossing my eyes, but I'm not. Another traumatic experience. Not the right medicine for me.

I leave the hospital on Trileptal. My new daily med. It makes me feel exhausted and nauseous. I'm told this will get better. I want to go rogue and stop taking it. But I can't drive until August 2017 right now. If I go rogue and have a seizure, that 6 months starts over. Is that worth it in a world that runs on gasoline?

I do not believe I need to be on anti-seizure medication forever. What I believe, what I perceive, does not really matter. Medicine matters. And my perceptions or feelings of how I experienced the psychosis, the seizures, the hospital are all put into question. Will and I are constantly getting *into dumb tiffs about the way I remember reality versus what he remembers. Who's right? Whose memories can be validated?*

Does it really matter?

III. WHAT I LEARNED ABOUT MYSELF

"When it rains, it pours."

Perseverance and humor

If you don't laugh, you'll cry.

You know those situations, when something is so dreadful that if you don't find the humor in it, you'll just destroy yourself dwelling on why it's so NOT funny? This is a huge way for me to "deal" with this dreadful predicament. I'll find as many things to laugh at as I can, always taking things seriously, but also laughing at the absurdity of life when we get TOO serious. I mean I KNOW I am seriously sick, but not laughing at the funny things doesn't make me better, it just makes life worse.

Not all cancer patients deal with things this way. I know I've made people uncomfortable with some of my jokes. I've always sort of had a dark, dry sense of humor, so it only seems natural to me that we would all join in on the "fun." I really don't want to intentionally make people uncomfortable. But I also feel like the person dealing with an illness is the one who gets to decide how to handle it.

For example, this whole "___ hair, don't care" thing is kind of popular right now. (Like ,"Long hair, don't care." I take it as "Yeah. I should probably get a haircut or style my hair, but what YOU think doesn't really matter to me, so I'll do what I want, thanks.")

I was at the airport and I saw a girl who was probably 12 wearing a shirt that said, "Gym hair, don't care." On the one hand, I liked it, because when I went to the gym, I often had gross, sweaty "gym hair" (and wore a t-shirt, sweats, and had a red face) and, indeed, did not care. On the other hand, I was wondering why a 12-year-old was hitting up a gym. Maybe she was talking about gym class. But I really hope, for the sake of young middle-schoolers everywhere, that she did not have a gym membership. Please play kickball on the playground.

Anyway, because I am judgmental sometimes and because I thought this situation a bit silly, I was telling my friend about this and she was like "omg, you should get that t-shirt and wear it around." The irony being that I had a shaved head and very little hair to speak of. I thought this idea was very, very funny. Because things like this totally make me laugh at my predicament. How ridiculous. How absurd.

I also really enjoy being semi-flip and sarcastic with my oncologist. To his credit, he knows this now and deals with me as I am. On one of the early visits we had after confirming I had cancer again we had to talk about what the plan was moving forward. There was a flyer in the little room we were in that had a very serious looking doctor with his arms crossed on it and said, "Hope is not a plan." This also cracked me up. I mean, that's true, but how brutal! The people coming in and out of that office are hopeful every day, and that's what keeps them rocking!

So, after Dr. Graber got through all of his thoughts and basically told Will and me about what treatment looked like moving forward, he said something along the lines of, "Does that all make sense to you?"

I just looked at him, pretty blank-faced, and said, "Sounds good. Because, you know, hope is not a plan."

He looked a little confused for a sec. I pointed at the sign and he started cracking up.

"I know," he said, "that sign is so horrible, right?"

Room for humor. I need that.

Humor is closely related to perseverance for me. It's how I keep going each day, in spite of the many challenges. Knowing that this whole experience is a ridiculous part of being human helps me see the humor in the everyday challenge and struggle of being alive—cancer or no cancer. And we all just do it, every day. One foot in front of the other, with humor or not.

There is the idea in the comedy community of punching up and punching down—that making fun of the little guy, or the marginalized, isn't very funny. It's (ONE) reason why rape jokes aren't funny. I think there needs to be another term for "punching across," which is what we should call it when a comedian makes us laugh because they are good at making fun of themselves and at how absurd it is to be human. I think Ellen Degeneres is very good at punching across.

It's good to take things seriously, because sometimes things are really serious. But I hope that more people than not choose humor over seriousness. There is so much to cry about in everyday human life. It seems especially important to find the things to giggle at, joke about, or just give a wry little smile to in our day-to-day endeavors. Plus, you can't get anything done if you're just crying the whole time.

Identity

Who are we? How much of who we are is our decision and how much of it is out of our control?

Certainly, we make choices all along the way that help define who we are. We have our hobbies, our friends, our clothes, and the music we listen to. But even much of that is decided by our upbringing and our peers.

You could always just ignore ALL of the outside influences and do what you love. That's probably the best option. But that takes a lot of strength and courage for most.

We also might change what we love in an instant or over time. And people DO completely change up their image and identity. Everyone needs space to do that. If we follow what we love, any change we make is more "'authentic" to our true selves. So, how much of authenticity is personal and how much of it can only be determined by external influences?

I've asked myself these questions quite a bit. On one hand, I've felt that I can totally decide how to deal with my identity as a young person with cancer. But I just as often feel completely helpless in this endeavor. I am not in control of many parts of my life, so living my truth doesn't always seem possible.

It was all so much easier the first time around. Having and treating cancer was all so fast. I could more easily put it behind me, thinking it was a "Well, THAT happened" situation. I'd move on, be just as much of a lost twenty-something as I was before. I had questions about how to accurately tell the story of my first experience with cancer, but for the most part, it became less and less relevant to my life. It became a distant thing, a thing that always lurked in the shadows, but never really came out to play.

Occasionally, I'd have some sort of "trigger moment." When I was teaching in a GED program for homeless students there was a girl in my class who, unfortunately, most of us knew to be an epic and perpetual liar. Once, she claimed to have brain cancer. It put me on edge to hear her say that to get some attention. I couldn't even talk to her and had to call on my co-teacher to deal with it. That was an odd experience, because I knew my students, knew they lied, and thought I could deal with it all. Apparently, traumatic experiences can induce hidden, emotional pain. Gee, who'd have thought?

Of course, I don't want cancer to define me. I don't WANT to be "that sick person who had to deal with it all so young." I don't like it when people think, "Well, she has cancer, so let's just talk about her health." How boring. But I also identify with this illness and its tribulations more than I ever did after I had it the first time. It's tough because I don't WANT it to define me, but I also know that it has shaped my life and perspectives in a way that I can't deny. And all of my deficiencies make a lot more sense if people know it's 'cause of brain cancer.

I struggle with not wanting to acknowledge my disease and also wanting the world to just know. That's right, people. Cancer is real and shitty, even in young, healthy-seeming people. We all know it's the worst, but many of us don't experience that first or even second-hand and I want people to know that I'm fucking strong.

You can never know someone's experiences just by looking at them, but I have always felt like I come off as a pretty nurtured suburban girl who has little insight into struggle. And sure, that's true of me in a lot of ways and I am grateful for all of the gifts life has given me. But despite my cushy upbringing, I know hard times. Like, really hard times. So, if you think I have nothing to offer or no perspective to understand adversity, then you don't know me very well.

Here I am, stuck with this conundrum: What is my identity? Am I a cancer survivor/someone with cancer? Or am I a strong woman who works to ignore her illness and see it for what it is—a shitty situation that no one could predict or control? Is it possible to be both?

I think it is. I can't deny the lessons I've learned or the experiences I've had. I used to be a pretty upbeat person. I was always down for that last drink, always ready for an all-nighter to finish that paper. I was very active and ready for that quick quip. Right now, I am a sleepy, confused, somewhat dour, sick person who can just barely take a long walk WITH A WALKER and who can't speak well enough to make a quick quip (part of my disability makes it difficult for me to form words). How does one reconcile these two identities?

I have some (amazing) friends who are definitely of the "Anyone can do anything" mindset. I love this, because they are the type of people who DO do (heehee) what they want. They pursue something with full steam, despite fears of change or failure. It's awesome. And inspiring. But I just can't help but think to myself, "Well, sometimes anyone CAN'T do ANYTHING."

That's what having cancer makes me feel. Sure, I'd love to learn how to rock climb, but I can't do that right now. I'd love to go on more hikes, but I can barely walk on my own, let alone climb a steep mountain with rocks. This isn't me being pessimistic—just realistic about what I can actually do on my own. I think when people say "Anyone can do anything," they really mean "Anyone with health, money, and time can do anything." If you're missing even one, you start to notice your limitations.

So this brings me back to identity. How much of it is in reaction to external happenings and how much of it is internal decisions and desires?

I suppose it's always a bit of both. It gets a little too philosophical for me to try to analyze the effects of nurture and nature on our psyches. But how does each pull on and affect the others?

I know these are not questions just for cancer patients, but like probably never before, this disease has really got me asking...

Who am I?

Spirituality

I didn't quite find Jesus or God through this experience, BUT cancer and my impending marriage came together in such a way that I really do feel as if I had a spiritual awakening.

Maybe that sounds all hippy dippy, and/or getting dunked in the ocean while others chant in the background. But it wasn't any of those things. It was only SLIGHTLY enhanced by prescribed drugs/the semi-psychotic break I had on said prescribed drugs. So maybe I have more insight into people who have spiritual awakenings on acid or shrooms or whatever else floats their boat. I would NOT suggest steroids. It doesn't feel very good.

Anyway. The awesome, wonderful officiant at our wedding, Anna McKinley (longtime family friend/spiritual guide), asked each of us to write something to her about our spirituality. That was something I had already been thinking about/seeking in my life since leaving home.

I grew up in a wonderful Episcopal church with my mom and it was a great community, I just could never quite get behind the whole Holy Trinity, Son of God stuff. And the idea of "A God." The Episcopal church is really quite cool about accepting that other people believe in other Gods, and I'm totally cool with that, too. Faith is (not) a fact. I'm actually okay with anybody believing what they want as long as they don't harm others or try to foist their faith upon others or do anything that I deem as generally fucked up (racist, sexist, classist, exclusionary, manipulative, you get it). My general motto is, "You do you." ESPECIALLY around religious beliefs.

So, basically, I was forced to put into words (first to Will, then to Anna) what my general beliefs are. And then while I was going through this psychotic break it all really came together for me. What I came up with is some combination of a YouTube video called "The Symphony of Science" and a graduation speech given in 2005 by

David Foster Wallace called *This is Water*. I suggest you use the powers of the internet to look them both up.

And then my friend Scottie said something to me about how in your 29th year your Saturn is returning, which means all sorts of transitions in your life (value neutral), and how much that was ringing true for me. I was going through this tough disease; I'd just started a new job that I LOVED, which may have been related to my career trajectory in a way I did not predict; I was getting MARRIED in July. It was just a lot of things.

So I started to look at astrology in a new light. I mean, I still think it's hit or miss and you can't just read a shitty newspaper horoscope and really plan your day around it, but I think there's something there.

I've always had trouble falling asleep. When I was a kid, my mom rubbed my back every night until I fell asleep and we said prayers together. This is something I still do. But now, "I pray to the universe (or Gaia) my soul to keep." And Will doesn't rub my back because he falls asleep in 5 minutes because he has the clearest conscience of anyone I know. But my spirituality is some combination of science and energy—because I BELIEVE in that idea. We are all connected—to each other, the earth, and the stars. I mean, guys, "WE'RE MADE OF STAR STUFF."

So, when I start praying about my family, I no longer think about just sending them good energy (though that, too). I also imagine my grandparents, all deceased, each up there as a star, just shining their light down on me a little brighter when they know I need it or if I ask for it. Because I think we all go back to the basics—we all become stars. When I think of the heavens, I think of the actual stars and the universe.

I also really like a saying I saw that said, "When you wish upon a star... that star is dead, just like your dreams." It's so brutally honest.

It made me laugh. Sometimes (all of the time), faith isn't based on logic.

This Is Water, just feels like a good motto to live by: Just give people the benefit of the doubt (or the Benny of the D, as Will and I affectionately call it). You literally never know where a stranger is coming from or what they're going through.

Sure, sometimes people are just jerks. And sometimes WE'RE not our best selves and WE'RE just jerks. But isn't the world a better place if we all just give each other a little grace? A little grace to mess up, or cut us off in traffic, or steal our parking spot, or, I don't know... the list goes on. I mean, don't get me wrong, I'm an angry driver. I am cussing other people out in a totally unnecessary manner. But I am alone in my car. They can't hear me. I don't seek them out for a confrontation. And I know most people don't, either.

The best Christians, Muslims, Jews, Hindus, Buddhists, Sikhs, and whatever else (I know there's more, I've just exhausted my knowledge of the major ones) live with love and patience for their neighbor. And understand that others live differently.

So that's the best I've got. It might sound kind of spacey or be ridiculous to base my spirituality on an auto-tuned YouTube video, but there's a reason I have come back to these two things over and over again in my life. They resonate with me. Really strongly. And if they don't resonate with you or you've already found what does, that's cool! I'm just sharing!

Like ANOTHER favorite YouTube video of mine explains, "Worry 'bout yo'self." (But only after you've carefully considered others' feelings, please.)

Public Presence

I'm pretty obvious-looking: I'm wearing an eye patch (to help with double vision); I'm usually in a wheelchair; and I can't smile, even at babies and animals (what kind of monster doesn't smile at babies and puppies? THIS kind of monster! The kind that can't smile!)

Long story short—my public persona does not often reflect what I'm actually feeling.

Little kids, who I mostly appreciate because they're so unapologetic and they so don't care what you look like, stare at me a lot in the streets. This I understand. It makes me sad, because I really like kids, so I want to be approachable, but I get it. I am a strange looking human that they don't understand. They have not been taught a world that includes humans like me. Maybe they've been taught not to stare at disabled people or people of other races than them, but a sort-of-"normal"-looking lady with an eye patch, no facial expressions, and her bottom lip just hanging down? What do they do with that? They're staring at me 'cause they're learning. And they want to be sure I'm not a monster that they should run away from. *Not yet, kiddies! Muahahah!*

Here's a fun story: I was in line at a carousel (this is when I still walked with a cane) where my then-two-year-old niece was fully enjoying herself, while the little girl next to me, about five, was just staring at me with such confusion and curiosity I almost talked to her. Her face was priceless. I wish I had a picture, because it was hilarious.

When adults stare at me, I want to punch them in the face. I get it, we all stare, sometimes involuntarily, it's human nature. But if you're above the age of 16, you should know better. Get your shit together. Turn away. Don't tell your friends to look at the strange person with a walker and an eye patch.. (I don't totally hate the public yet, but they're testing me….) One time a GROWN adult stranger passed me on the sidewalk and said, "Arrrr, matey!" in response to, I believe, my eye patch. I don't know if he was kidding or if he assumed I was kidding. Either way, we all know what happens when we assume….

Anyway, point is, I am not in control of who I am in public and many of us are not. I also have learned that we live in a very Ableist society. Our sidewalks are very bumpy and there are fewer curb cuts than there should be. I prefer using a wheelchair over a walker, because even though the walker would exercise my legs more and help more with balance, people are nicer and more helpful to someone in a wheelchair. I think it's because it's more obvious and because our society teaches us that walkers are for people who did something TO THEMSELVES and wheelchairs are for people who had something done TO THEM. People in wheelchairs DESERVE help. People with walkers don't.

I'm very lucky to have a strong husband who heaves me over the curbs I can't get myself over, but not everyone has that. Part of me gets it: You build your world to accommodate 75 percent of the people, not 25 percent. But a curb cut (or a ramp, or an elevator) doesn't seem that hard.

What does this have to do with communication, you ask? I'm getting there, I promise. I think people pay less attention to those who are disabled. Actually, I'll amend that to say that people pay less WANTED or NEEDED attention to those who are disabled. Sure, people love to gawk and stare and be annoyed when you take longer to get on the bus, but mostly they would prefer that you were not in their way. That you would just go away or act like everyone else.

This is where communication becomes important. When you are disabled you have to be willing to communicate your needs more, be more willing to say "excuse me," and be more willing to ask someone what the best way to get inside is or where the bathroom is or whatever. You have to learn to communicate better, with strangers and with loved ones who are just trying to be helpful.

It's really hard, but being straightforward about what you need and why you need it is just best for everyone. It's especially hard for females, who have been taught our whole lives that being straightforward is "bitchy," and for Seattleites, who are the kings of passive aggression.

I have not mastered it, for sure, but I think we are all probably better off if we say what we mean and mean what we say. If we can offer a solution to a problem, all the better.

Asking for help

There is a famous story in my family: I am two. I am attentively watching *Sesame Street* so my mom, who has been folding laundry (shoutout to all of the moms out there for their multi-tasking skills!), decides she can take ten seconds to run the folded laundry upstairs. She comes back down to an open front door and me, halfway down the block, telling our neighbor, "I go park."

I think the reason this story is so popular with my parents (besides just being funny) is because a) it shows that I've ALWAYS been an independent bitch and it's not entirely their fault; and b) asking for help when I clearly need help (like being two but wanting to go to the park) is hard for me.

For one, I hate putting other people out. I know on some level this is stupid. People love to help and I know that when I can be helpful to someone it feels AMAZING. Any good deed is partially selfish—that doesn't undo its goodness, it's just true: Being good to others feels good. I think it's proof that we're meant to be nice to one another. We are biologically programmed to feel good when we do good by others. That's kind of awesome.

For another, I am fiercely independent and stubborn (and a bit of a control freak), so asking for help is admitting I can't do something on my own and that whomever I am asking can have full control over how a thing gets done. Asking for help is not only admitting I am not fully capable, it's also relinquishing control over how I do something. Control is a big thing in the cancer world (as you'll read more of later). That's something you can grant your loved ones with cancer: control.

I've had to learn how to express my needs. I've had to learn that it's okay to be selfish. It sounds like I'm really talking myself up. "Oh, I'm so selfless. Oh, I hate putting people out." But I really have had to teach myself what it means to ask for help when you need it, because when you don't, you fall and break your shoulder. (I know this because I did exactly that, trying to be independent and not asking for help. So. Worth. It!).

Maybe all of these things are just planets that orbit the sun of identity. (I tried to think of a better metaphor than that but couldn't come up with one.) A huge part of my identity is that I'm someone who doesn't need help. I was the kind of person who took the stairs even when there was an escalator.

Now I am someone who needs help. I am someone who never takes the stairs. Learning to communicate my needs is something I'm STILL working on and probably always will be.

Appearance

When you are ill, your appearance changes. The biggest thing with cancer is that people often lose their hair.

The first time around, the chemotherapy and radiation left me completely bald. This time around, it has meant shorter hair, slower growth, and more thinning. Before all of this, I had very long (too long), thickish locks. It was nice hair.

I used to really miss it and it took me a while to get over that part of myself, ESPECIALLY as I planned a wedding and all of the bridal styles were these incredible updos that I just didn't have the hair for. Ultimately, I love how my stylist did my hair. It was unique and regal and not any way I would have expected! She did a great job, even if it wasn't what I always imagined.

The thing I hated so much about being bald wasn't necessarily the bald part (I look kinda good bald, if I say so myself), it was the public declaration that "I'm sick! Yeah, you're right, it's cancer!" that I really didn't like.

When I was bald, I had a female friend be like, "Do you want me to shave my head in solidarity?"

This is so nice, but I was like, "NO! First of all, you have beautiful hair, and second of all, IT WON'T MAKE ME FEEL BETTER TO HAVE A BUNCH OF BALD PEOPLE AROUND ME!!"

This leads me to one of my #unpopularcanceropinions, and that opinion is that solidarity efforts are silly. I know they come from a place of goodness, but shaving your head doesn't mean you understand the pain of cancer, and a bunch of bald people doesn't make cancer go away. It feels like that kind of "solidarity effort" is all about the person without cancer. I know some of these efforts raise awareness of the disease and funds for research, but I might argue that these funds could be raised without the unnecessary baldness.

Anyway, society sets all of these insane expectations of women and what brides are supposed to look like. Duh, we know this, but my cancer has turned me into someone I don't totally recognize when I look in the mirror. That is weird and hard. I used to feel pretty, which according to everything I've been taught is a huge part of what makes my existence worthwhile.

Again, I think appearance and cancer have a lot to do with control and choice. I can CHOOSE not to shave my armpits. I can CHOOSE to cut off all of my hair. I cannot choose to smile at the stranger passing, or laugh at your joke, or wear my contacts because I feel like it (part of my dysphasia is an inability to close my eyes all the way, which = very dry eyes).

Part of having cancer has been learning how to feel pretty again, which was hard enough BEFORE cancer!

System navigation

Cancer teaches you a lot about hospitals and a lot about insurance. And a lot about other things you don't care about.

First of all, if there was ever a case for universal health care, it's cancer (I don't think there really needs to be a "case," it seems like a major "duh" to me). Cancer is damn expensive! An MRI alone, a scan that I need every two months, costs thousands of dollars! Thank Gaia I have good health insurance, because otherwise I'd be cookin' meth with my friend Jesse.*

What do people do when they don't have a job and aren't married to someone with good health insurance? Declare bankruptcy, I guess. Which has to be great for the economy.

Cancer is not something you choose or something that only happens to "unhealthy" people. Hell, I was 23 and probably in some

*I do not have any friends named Jesse, and I would never make drugs to pay my medical bills. This is, you guessed it, another pop culture reference. ("Breaking Bad.")

of the best shape of my life when I first had cancer. Cancer and many other illnesses/conditions are not choices. If I had my choice, I'd be living without cancer, walking everywhere, taking the bus. This lack of choice is why we need a system that works for everyone, because not everyone has the same choices as you.

One good thing about cancer is that I have become very adept at dealing with systems and red tape, and at knowing when to go around that red tape and when to just be patient. Often patience is the answer, unfortunately. Cancer has definitely made me a more patient person. (Which I guess is a good thing since patience is a virtue and blah, blah, blah....)

Some things I've learned about systems: 1) You catch more flies with honey and 2) The squeaky wheel gets the grease.

What do I mean by these things? Well, first, let's acknowledge what a weird expression "You catch more flies with honey" is. I don't want more flies! No one wants more flies! Except maybe spiders and they don't talk and use weird expressions (that we know of).

The point is, the person you are talking to likely has no impact on the system, but they might make your day better by transferring you to the right department or bringing up your issue in a meeting where someone who *can* do something is present, so BE NICE TO THAT PERSON. That person probably also has a shit job where stressed-out strangers yell at them all day about things they wish they could fix, but cannot.

And more than just to get something out of it, be nice to that person because they are a PERSON. With a little empathy, you can imagine that person is you. And you wouldn't want someone yelling at you all day about something over which you have no control.

And "the squeaky wheel gets the grease" means exactly what it sounds like: BE ANNOYING. Call a lot. E-mail all of the time. If you get an answer, and you don't like it but there's nothing more to be done or that person can do, then leave it alone. There's annoying and there's ANNOYING. Do not make others beat their heads against the wall, but make sure you get the attention you deserve. Sometimes that means being a little annoying. It always means be patient.

I've thought about putting this ability to navigate systems to work and becoming a social worker, but I'm not a good listener and there isn't enough money in the world to make me want to be a social worker. (And they definitely don't make all of the money in the world.) Big thanks to all you social workers out there. You probably don't hear this enough, but you are amazing.

Self-love/care

Self-love is real and important. It's especially important when you're fighting a disease. Mind over body, positivity over negativity. It's powerful and can affect how our bodies treat us or anything else inside of us.

I do think self-love is highly connected to appearance—you need to like what you see when you look in the mirror (or at least be content with it). But I also think self-love goes deeper than what you look like. I think self-love has a lot to do with liking WHO you are and the choices you make about who you want to be.

Cancer is a taker. In fact, there's not much that cancer gives you. I take that back. It gives you lots of things. It gives you anxiety. Frustration. Fear. Nausea. Loss of control. Nothing you want. Mostly, it takes things away from you, especially when it comes to your body and your self-esteem. Your self-love.

I haven't really worked out or been consistently active now for years. For some people, I suppose this is normal, but for me, it's a really long time. I am, and always have been, a very active person.

This lack of activity takes away my muscle, my strength, my weekly endorphin fix. And leaves me with a body and mind I don't recognize or even like.

The hardest thing is the lack of strength. I have always been a physically strong person. Able to carry a heavy box. Able to walk straight up a hill without having to stop for a breather. Able to hold a yoga pose for a long time, even as my muscles shake. But now, I feel like a weak person. I am strong in other ways, but I believe physical strength helped me stay and feel mentally strong. And where'd that go? Whoosh. Another thing lost to fighting cancer.

I've talked about my hair, but I will talk about it again. Sure, I just need to get over it. And mostly I am. I definitely WAS. Right now, I have very short, thin hair. It's easier. But I still miss long hair and all the creativity that comes with it. Even if I have long hair again, it will likely be thin.

Liking my long hair felt like a big part of self-love—to learn to focus on things I loved about myself and appreciate those things. I was beginning to do that again. Let go of the 2010 hair and be fine with the 2015/2016 hair. Whoosh.

Right now, I'm suffering from facial palsy. That means the nerves in your face that control your smile and your eyes (blinking or not) don't work. I currently cannot fully close my eyes. (I had gold weights surgically put under my eyelids, but they are still open a little bit.) Nor can I smile. Nor can I kiss. The whole bottom of my face just kinda hangs there like a dead fish or something. They think this is because there is cancer on my nerves. Or my nerves have been severely affected by radiation. Either cause is not good, although I suppose any cause that doesn't involve cancer is inherently better.

I liked my hair? I also liked my smile. I cannot smile any more. I don't feel I can fully express myself. I hate the person I see looking back at me. Supposedly, this will gradually get better. I really hope so. Because otherwise, whoosh! Right now, definitely whoosh!

What else? There can't be more. There is, but not a whole lot. My cancer was (is?) in my cerebellum, which controls balance, so I am quite unsteady on my feet. My left hand is also shaky and has a mind of its own. I let things just drop to the ground out of no choice of my own. Typing, which was always very fast for me, is laborious and slow. Walking alone is not really possible for me. This may improve. It might just be part of who I am now.

So, what is this other than a laundry list of complaints about all of the visibly physical ways this stupid disease has made me feel less like myself and more like a strange cloning attempt?

Well, it's that *and also* this rumination on self-love and what that really means. I've been working on self-love for a while now, trying to remind myself, especially, that our bodies are fading vessels and that who we ARE as people is what counts as beautiful and makes us US.

I think, though, no matter how beautiful someone is, they have to work through and come to terms with their physical presence. It's a big part of what people think and feel about you, whether we like it or not. This is especially true for women.

At the very least, I think we have to try to like (most days) what we present to the world and try to feel comfortable in our skin. That's what the movement is about, right? Taking selfies when we think we look hot. Putting on a new outfit and thinking "damn!" before walking out the door. Overall, appreciating ourselves.

This seems like an especially important time to learn to appreciate my evolving self. We all change. Cancer takes a whole lot, but ya know what else does? Time. Time abuses us all. And we must persist in finding the things we love. Or at least like.

"...*Even as I recognized that I had lost a little*
Of that connection between my eyes and hands.

But haven't I been losing shit all along? As we age,
Don't we all deteriorate? If I can't hit as many smashes
In table tennis or swish as many jump shots in basketball
Or write as many poems as I did before brain surgery,
Then so be it. I am alive! I am alive! I am alive!..."

(This is an excerpt from Sherman Alexie's most recent book *You Don't Have to Say You Love Me*, which is a memoir and very sad, but has many delightful things in it. This passage continues on, and ends beautifully.)

Self-care seems like the perfect companion of self-love. For love, we have to deem ourselves worthy of love and for care, we have to deem ourselves worthy of care. I won't pretend to know the chicken and the egg of it all, 'cause I don't. Cancer has helped me see how important taking care of ourselves is.

I get massages, acupuncture, and let my mom treat me to manicures and pedicures when she is here. You know, sometimes it just feels good to be taken care of.

I know that cancer gives me a lot more space to do these things—I don't have a job that demands my presence 40+ hours/week and I have no kids to feed or read to; I'm sick so lots of people pay for stuff and give me gifts (FYI, being sickly is NOT worth it)—but I think everyone needs to find a little bit of time in their life for self-care. Whether it's taking that nap you've been craving or something pricier, like getting massages twice/month (self-care looks different for everyone), I think taking a moment that is completely about US and OUR needs can be healthy.

When I was growing up, my mom got her nails done every two weeks by this woman named Rosemary who works out of her home and who watched me grow. I remember asking my mom once why she got a manicure every two weeks. She said, "I told myself that if I ever had steady income and could afford it, I would get a manicure every two weeks. Nice nails will be my thing." This was not a rich, unbusy lady—my mom was a teacher with two kids. But nice nails were her thing, damnit, and she definitely always had nice nails! When I was younger, I always saw this as an "I made it" sort of thing, and while I think that's part of it, I also think part of it is self-care.

So, as it turns out, I had a wonderful model for self-care, even if I didn't know it at the time. We can't take care of others if we don't take care of ourselves.

Youth

I think one reason young adult cancer is so hard, and I've touched on this a bit, is that it robs you of your youth. Old people are supposed to be sick, not young people. Young adults are supposed to be getting married or dating or drinking or dancing or finding their career, not learning how to use a walker or spending days with a caretaker.

One minute, I am the child who can't be trusted to do things on her own, the next minute I am the ignored old lady outside of the action who is hard to understand and can't hear well enough to follow what's going on.

I've had so much taken from me and one of the major things is my youth. I only get one chance to be young, there isn't a redo, and much of my youth has been defined by hospitals and tubes. I have to also remember that a good chunk of my youth is defined by coloring books, and bike rides, and cookie dough, and LOVE. 'Cause even though, RIGHT NOW sucks, I've been a pretty lucky duck in this one life.

#YOLO

Unfortunately, YOLO [an acronym for "You Only Live Once"] *was turned into a silly hashtag that is typically associated with (white) teenagers doing stupid things in the spirit of living life fully.*

Part of me is on board with this interpretation: There is only once in your life where you can duck* up and it's all probably going to be okay. Plus, when you're a teenager, you have no fear and should take risks. To a point.

I like to, jokingly, use this spirit of YOLO when I am doing something adults "shouldn't" do or when I do something out of character for me. You only live once has taken on special meaning to me right now: I better do the stuff I've always wanted to do now, while I still can. And while I physically cannot do some of it, I gotta do what I am able to do.

Like dye my hair a shocking, very unnatural red. Which I did. Like a week ago. 'Cause, you know, YOLO.

The other interpretation of YOLO could be that you only have one life, so you better take care of it. You better not smoke. You should wear sunscreen. Always have a seat belt on.

I think both interpretations are valid and needed at different times. I had a friend who is allergic to bees, and on a hike I was giving him a lot of shit about getting an EpiPen and he was all, "Well if that's how I'm gonna go, then so be it."

This made me laugh because it. Is. So. Stupid! It's like the worst interpretation of YOLO ever: taking a totally unnecessary risk because to NOT take it is mildly annoying and a slight inconvenience.

---

*"Duck" is how my phone has chosen to auto correct the "f" word.** I find this charming, so I rarely change it. It's just so ducking cute!

**Sometimes I am actually talking about a duck, like the animal. Turns out I actually talk about ducks a fair amount. *Duck!*

Yes, we only get one life and we should live it fully and the way we want to, but we should also try to protect ourselves where we can. Just existing is a risk. So we should take the risks that make existence worth it.

So, if you've always wanted to jump out of a plane, go sky diving.

'Cause... you know, YOLO.

IV. WHAT I LEARNED ABOUT OTHERS

"The grass is always greener...."

Before I launch into any specifics, I really want to emphasize that we all do our best. We all have lives and things going on and often kids that take up a lot of time and energy. There isn't much to say except, "I'm sorry," and, "This sucks." Although there are plenty of "wrong" things to say, like, "God has a plan for us all," or, "You're in God's hands now." Wasn't I always in his hands? And if this is part of the plan, then God is a shitty event planner.

I don't believe in God in THAT way (as you know), but I've come to appreciate most of these responses because TO THAT PERSON, the response IS meaningful. It means they were thinking about me, which is nice. Plus, I've only ever had one dumdum say the "plan" thing to me. I think we all recognize how little comfort that brings in hard times.

My point is that, in cancer (not to mention every other tough situation), we could all use a little grace and patience. It's hard and there is no clear right and wrong. We all just do our best.

My Community

I have been lucky to have an amazing community—of nurses, of therapists, of friends, of friends of friends, and even of animals! These are really important relationships that I've been lucky to grow during this time, but I'll say that, for me, they're not enough.

For me, a huge part of community is getting out there. Riding the bus. Living amongst the neighborhood characters.

One of my favorite moments from when I lived on Capitol Hill in Seattle happened at a music festival in our neighborhood. Will and I weren't actually attending the festival but it was a nice day, in the middle of a July afternoon, so we were sitting on a porch, having some drinks and people-watching. A guy from the festival was walking by and he was dressed as "Scarf Man".

Now, anyone who has ever been to a Seattle event knows Scarf Man. He is an old dude, with a beard, who often has his shirt off, and does a lot of scarf dancing as he encourages others to join him, mostly by throwing colorful scarves at them. So... a guy at the festival, dressed like Scarf Man, walks by where we are seated outside, and everyone around us starts yelling, "Hey, you aren't the real Scarf Man!" To which there was a symphony of, "Yeah!"'s.

Now, to me, that's community: People who don't know each other at all and maybe have nothing in common other than that they all live in Seattle, all reacting in the same way toward someone dressed as a local character.

You don't get that by staying at home, sitting on your couch, watching Netflix. But that's where I am most days, figuratively and literally. Community is knowing your neighbors and your neighborhood, even if that just means seeing the same people on the bus all of the time.

Cancer has meant that I have a very different community, a community of nurses and doctors and healthcare professionals. It is a very kind community, but I have to say it is not the community I would like to have.

This means I rely a lot on social media to feel connected to the world.

Social Media

I'm not the first person to see or write on the toxic nature of social media: It can be really terrible. Everyone is projecting their best life all of the time. It's not always a fabrication, that's just when we take pictures: when we are succeeding or having fun! We don't often take pictures or post when we are sad or lying on the couch for days on end. Most of us, DO get sad or angry, we just don't tend to tell the world about it. That can feel so isolating, like everyone is having fun without you. Or you should be prettier, skinnier, hiking more, eating more kale, or whatever. By the way, I know there are many who disagree with me, but kale is disgusting,

Social media can also normalize something that would, generally, seem strange. This can be great because it means that a whole bunch of "outcasts" can find "their people" and connect with them. I've made connections on social media this way, even if sometimes brief, with other young adults with cancer, as well as with people in my neighborhood.

The flip side—and I've thought about this since social media began really blowing up—is that negative behavior can be reinforced. I remember reading an article about bulimics and how they had a whole group online to tell others how to do it, how to hide it, before and after photos, etc. A really bad thing that would typically be noticed by friends and family was given a space to normalize and I think that's really concerning.

We put ourselves in bubbles of agreement anyway, and it's always our job to monitor that for ourselves, social media or not. I do believe that things like Instagram and Facebook are negative as much as we let them be negative. They can also be really great.

I say all of this because I've never been one to be on my phone a lot. (I didn't get a "smart" phone until 2015 or 2016 and if it weren't for how helpful the camera and maps are and how much joy emojis bring me, I would just go back.) Yet, now that cancer has taken so much from me (like typing, and my eyesight, and my speech and my hearing) I am buried in my phone A LOT. Things like Facebook and Instagram are my connection to the world. A way to get away, mentally, when I

physically can't. It's also why I like tv and movies so much.
They are a way to get away.

I do believe that we need to be more present in our lives,
but sometimes our lives suck. And we just wanna get away.
Sometimes this means social media.

I guess what I'm trying to say about community is that you often get what you give. (I think there is a Beatles song related to that idea, so—see?—triteness CAN be inspiring.) When you're stuck inside all of the time, our communities are often not what we imagined or prefer.

Friendship

Cancer has been wonderful in showing me that I have more friends than I thought I had, and it has shown me that adult friendship is just HARD.

I knew this, but cancer solidified it for me. It takes a certain level of effort to be a more or less GOOD friend, and many of us don't have the time or energy for it. There are also fewer friend-finding opportunities like school and clubs and extracurriculars, as you get older. Adult friendship can sometimes feel forced and less organic. That has been ESPECIALLY true as I've been house-bound and the coolest thing I have to offer is a movie partner or someone to binge Netflix with (which is mostly a solo activity… or like a "Netflix and chill" activity).

Generally, who I consider to be my closest friends fall into three categories: Those who hide, those who cling, and those who somehow get it just right.

I will say that 95 percent of people fall into the category of getting it right, more or less. And when I say "right," I mean appropriate to our relationship and what I need from them, not what THEY need from me. And before anyone worries that they fall into a certain category and so I am "mad" at them, I want to be clear: I am not mad at anyone, but I do want to explain what these categories mean.

1. Those who hide

This means exactly what it sounds like (or doesn't sound like... haha): Radio Silence. From people I KNOW have time for a text or email.

No word. Nothing. No checking in. And I know there are many reasons for this: Life is hard and we all got lives; insecurity about what to say; it's too much and it triggers you; or you just don't care that much that my current life is a living hell.

I want and choose to believe it's not because you don't care. Because if *I* actually care about it, that means we once DID care A LOT about each other. And I know I said I'm not mad, but silence is unacceptable and selfish. Maybe you need to be selfish right now. Maybe you don't know how much things DO suck—A THING YOU WOULD KNOW IF YOU EVER CHECKED IN.

But like I said, I'm not mad at you. I may be frustrated, but I know that life is short and holding on to frustration is not helpful for ANYONE, least of all, me. If you are feeling like, "Oh, I've been so silent for so long, I better just stick with it..." then please, please don't think that way. I WANT to hear from you. I don't want it to be too late before you show that you cared.

2. Those who cling

These are the people who overdo it. These people think of me as worse than I am and are pretty sure I am dying tomorrow. They want to visit NOW. They reach out, inappropriately, even though we were never friends. They come out of the woodwork and decide that I NEED them. They do not understand my needs and they are very overwhelming.

I know that it often "comes from love" or what THEY perceive as love, but I think there is also some desire to be close to tragedy. Or maybe I'm just cynical. I'm definitely cynical.

3. Those who manage to get it just "right"

Like I said, "right" is relative and what works for me and what I need changes, which I think makes this especially hard.

Generally, those who have gotten it "just right" have treated me like they always have, with the understanding that I cannot be who I always was or want to be. Or they have given the right support to Will. This has looked like many different things, but often just means listening: listening to what I say in any moment, listening to Will as he struggles through what it means to take care of a sick wife, listening to what we need, right then. And responding, if they can, to fill that need.

A great example I can think of was my desire to get a pet: I really wanted to hang out with an animal. I needed unconditional love like only an animal can provide. And I have read that animals are a good thing for recovery.

Will is allergic to cats. So a dog was really the best option for us, but a dog is a lot of work, and that likely meant a lot more work for Will (since I'm already more work than he expected). So a friend of ours, we'll call him Gary, arranged with a friend of HIS to have weekly visits with her incredibly well-behaved dog, Javi.

Javi is amazing. And Gary helps out by dropping him off, picking him up, and being generally available should he be needed at any point during the day. THAT was being a really good friend in so many ways: providing me support, providing Will support, and really listening. Like I said, most people I know fall into this category of getting it "right" and I'm so, so lucky they do.

I may not feel as connected to the community of Beacon Hill as I felt to the community of Capitol Hill, but I have seen the people in my life show up time and time again to help me out, show me patience, and make feel strong when I've felt low. I have special people from different walks of life, who mean the world to me, and many of these people I knew long before I could walk!

Husband

Phew, let's talk about friendship! Your husband should be your best friend. You should be attracted to one another—like, you should definitely find someone who would make you swipe right.* And I think sex and attraction are an important part of a relationship. But you should ALSO be with someone who "gets" you and who you "get."

---

*Pop reference. On the dating app Tinder, moving your finger to the right over a thumbnail image means you find that person appealing. To the left…not so much.

I have always thought that you need to find "the same kind of asshole you are." And I think, by this, I have always meant someone who is on your level: someone who makes you laugh and who you make laugh, someone who knows why you did something or why you like what you like, and someone who both accepts you as you are but also pushes you to be better.

Life is HARD, illness or not, and you better attach yourself to someone who makes it feel less hard and sees you as a human. We all make mistakes and we all poop. If you think you are walking away from your relationship without the other person hearing you fart or using the bathroom after you've pooped, then I really think you're delusional (or your house is too big and you have too many bathrooms). When you are sick, you will likely not feel sexy. You'll talk about poop and pee and blood in a way that you never have before. If you are with someone you aren't comfortable talking about those things with, then don't get sick. I guess that's why vows have the whole "in sickness and in health" thing.

I guess, in many ways, my relationship with my husband is very much tied to my appearance. Cancer has really changed the way I look, and if my husband didn't love me for something other than my looks (and I'm telling ya, I was a pretty hot little number when we got together), we'd be in real trouble here. Cancer has taken away all of my best physical features.

One thing they don't talk about, and I can see why, is that you will likely not feel very sexy during illness. I mean, somebody else picks out my underwear and cleans up my poop. There are no secrets—which I think is a HUGE part of sexiness. Sure, you want to be with someone who KNOWS you're a human, but you also want the opportunity to keep them as distanced from that part of your humanity as possible.

Will is good at making me feel beautiful and sexy even when I feel my ugliest/least sexy. And he is good at acknowledging the things he DOES miss, without making me feel bad about it, which I really appreciate because pretending I'm all the same or that I look really good is just a lie.

"Things change, right?" he has said to me on more than one occasion.

There's another thing Will always says, and that I have found useful: "We are on the same team."

This is a great way of putting it. He might be playing forward and I might be playing keeper, but at the end of the day, we want the same thing: to win.

You don't blame your forwards when you have zero goals, or tell the keeper they are rubbish when a goal goes in. (Sorry, I get all British when I talk about foo... er, soccer.) At least you shouldn't. Because you are a team. That keeper already feels worse than they should. Same goes for those forwards.

Point is, no one is going to play their role right 100 percent of the time. We all need practice and patience and grace.

Family and Family friends

Hopefully you can realize the importance of these people without getting sick, but no one will be there for you like family, and the adults in your life who are like family. I sort of knew this already. But cancer has really shown me how supportive these people are, and in confronting death and identity and all that, I have really seen how much I would miss these people and how important they have been in shaping who I am.

I have a godmother who sends me a card, the cheesier the better, every month. She has sent me soft and warm things (some of which have become my favorites), and has really been there for my mom, when she has needed her most.

I always knew this person was very important to me, but not being someone who seeks God all that often, a person "responsible for my religious upbringing"—which is one of the things a godparent traditionally is (I think a more modern definition is just like a close friend or someone who doesn't already have a title, but that you want in your child's life)—may not have seemed as important as they actually are.

This person has been a FANTASTIC godmother, never forgetting me at Christmas, or on my birthday, but she, and other family friends, is tied to who I am in a way that I could not see before I got ill. Cancer can bring people out of the woodwork and sometimes, those are people you never meant to put in the woodwork in the first place.

I have said there is nothing like family, and I believe that to be true. If you are lucky enough to come from a good family, these people can almost always be counted on for a pick-me-up or moral support. In the eyes of my parents, I will always be their baby. What do you do when your baby is sick? You take care of that baby. In this case, the person with cancer is the baby, doesn't matter if you're 29 or 92 (though if you are 92 and your parents are still alive, then holy shit! Stop reading this book, you've got GREAT genes, you'll be FINE).

I can't really say what a family SHOULD do if a young adult in their family falls ill, besides shower the sick person with love and treat them like an adult (they may be young, but they ARE an adult, after all), but I can say one thing they should definitely NOT do: trash any part of the care team.

I'm guessing this ill person spends a lot of time (read: more than family members) with these people, and would probably seek a better care team if they thought things would be better somewhere else. The sick person needs to trust their care team in order to get better. A family member can be as frustrated behind the loved one's back as they need to be (because cancer is really effing frustrating), but to their face, the sick person needs to hear about the care team's accolades, not how they have messed up. (Of course, if you think someone is being taken advantage of or not being served by their team, then you should definitely have an intervention and make them see someone else.)

I am nothing if not the product of my people. I am a deeply loyal person and I take friendship and relationship very seriously. I like to think this is a good thing, but it can mean you get burned—a lot. You can care more about someone than they care about you. Your group of close friends is small and you don't end up with a bustling social life. But when you DO find someone you connect with, they are usually a diamond in the rough. (I can't say that phrase without thinking about the Disney version of Aladdin—early 1990s. Anyone else?)

Cancer has made me see how important those people are and how much I am me because of them—all of them, my husband, my community, ALL of my friends, and my family.

V. WHAT I'VE LEARNED ABOUT CANCER

"When the going gets tough
the tough get going."

Loss of control

The biggest thing with cancer—a "duh," maybe, to everyone but me—is loss of control. You feel betrayed by your own body and like things just keep HAPPENING to you rather than you deciding what you want your body to do. I think this is probably extra true for young adults who are supposed to be healthy and in control of their bodies.

I find myself wanting control over things I never cared about before, and realizing areas of my life that I've had to let others control that I never would have thought about before. A good example of this is my dresser. Before, when I was headed into work, I picked out my own outfits and I put all of my clothes away. Now, I mostly don't do any of that. Will or the caretaker choose what I will wear (often with guidance from me, of course) and put away my clothes. I have always had a very specific way of organizing my clothes and it can drive me a little crazy to watch others choose their own systems and ruin mine, but it's not something worth holding onto so I just...

...Give it up.

Another thing that cancer can teach you to relinquish is control over your own body. You often have to just do what you're told. Give blood 'cause someone said so. Get poked because you're getting a scan and that's just part of it. Sure, you can refuse anything you want along the way, but maybe it will mean death. What kind of control is that?

Ultimately, I feel I have lost control of the way in which I want to live. And maybe it's all an illusion. Maybe we don't actually have control of anything, but I feel painfully aware of the loss of that illusion. I feel attached to the Pacific Northwest because I feel attached to my medical team. I LOVE the Pacific Northwest but I wonder what sort of choices I would make if I had more control over my life. Would I choose to stay anyway? Would it FEEL different because of that?

Another thing I think about often is control over my career. At a time when everyone is figuring out what they do for a living, I'm just trying to live. And what I WANT to do, I feel like I can't.

When you have cancer you lose control, from the mundane to the really important. We are more than our jobs and more than our bodies, but when you don't get to decide that, they feel like everything.

Silver Linings

There are definitely benefits to being sickly (something I like to call #cancerperks) and there better be, because being sick suuuucks, in so many ways.

Generally, people are nicer to you if you visibly have cancer (like when you are bald - which doesn't always mean you are ill!) or if/when they find out you have cancer. You get to play the Cancer Card when you don't want to do something or something doesn't go your way. You want to be careful with this, though, because it really loses its power if you use it too much.

It IS nice to have people do things for you just 'cause, but I was lucky to already have that. And be more in control of it. I think the biggest "silver lining" of losing things is that you get to realize what really matters to you. You learn where you are willing to compromise and where you aren't. For me, what really matters is people, experiences, and independence. I've had to make a LOT of compromises around these things and part of being sick is having to decide where compromise is worth it. It's not always very clear, especially when we're talking about relationships, but it seems like it happens a lot: deciding when medicine is worth the risk, deciding when to get a caregiver and when you'll be fine on your own, and deciding what is best for you versus what is best for others.

That brings me to another silver lining that I didn't mention: Cancer has given me the opportunity to practice all of the things I am worst at! It has shown me the value in listening when we might want to talk. The importance of silence for everyone, every now and then, and patience, always. It has helped me practice what I preach, in many ways. I like to think I was headed more in that direction as I aged *anyway,* but I suppose if I have to have an illness like this, I might as well look for the #cancerperks.

Babies!

Let's address the elephant in the room. I mean, you can't get cancer in your late twenties without talking about pregnancy. It just seems natural for anyone, male or female but ESPECIALLY for a female since men can have babies until they're like 100. Ew.

Let's be clear: No one is certain that I wouldn't be able to get pregnant in the future. But SHOULD I get pregnant has a pretty clear answer and the answer is no. I have been twice radiated and undergone multiple rounds of chemo, some of it VERY strong, and any future child I had would likely have a very difficult life. I know this is a concern with ANY pregnancy, chances are just really high for me.

Anyway, this was never a big thing for me—I always felt like there were so many kids out there that needed homes anyway, and I know adoption is no picnic but neither is pregnancy! Adopted kids are better for the earth and would be better for my body. All that stuff. Then two things... nope, three things... happened that really changed my perspective:

1) I saw the movie *Lion* and one of those adopted kids is super messed up and traumatized;

2) I married a really awesome person who I would love to have a kid with; and,

3) everyone and their mothers started having babies.

Seems the twenties are when everyone gets married and the thirties are for children.* Two of our friends have kids, two just recently had kids, my cousins (who are near to my age—one is EXACTLY my age, as in we were born in the same year) just had kids, and four of our friends have announced recent pregnancies. Oh, and my sister-in-law is having a (second) child! Babies, babies everywhere! (But not a drop to drink! *Rime of the Ancient Mariner?* Anyone?)

I don't know if it's baby fever, everyone around me, or my illness, but I'm starting to feel this desire to be pregnant.

Don't get me wrong, at the very beginning of all of this, this was brought up as a concern. (If you or a loved one is going to undergo any chemotherapy or radiation, this, at least, merits a conversation no matter their sex.) I went to a fertility clinic, where I felt more like a client than a patient, was treated kind of rudely, and I ultimately decided not to go that route.

One, it was going to mean more delays in treatment and more pokes and prods that I didn't feel like dealing with. Second, they really wanted to freeze not just eggs but also embryos (fertilized eggs). Will and I had been together for, like, nine years, but he had JUST proposed. Asking him to fertilize an egg so that we could MAYBE have a baby together in the future felt like too much.

---

*In true millennial style, many of my close friends are not married and I'm 31!

Plus, what if I died? Then what? Does a surrogate bring me back to life through a new baby? It seemed like a lot of questions to answer without proper information. I said no. Not because of monetary cost—my brother offered money, the place itself offered a generous discount to cancer patients—but out of a different kind of cost: an emotional cost that I can't accurately calculate.

And sure there are things I regret (hindsight IS 20/20), but this is not one of them. It wasn't the right thing to do. I still don't feel like it was the right thing to do.

There is a part of me that wants to experience pregnancy… like it's a rite of passage that women go through, often together. But I know a lot of people that I think of as strong, tough women who don't have kids, don't plan to have kids, or can't have kids for a variety of reasons. Does that make them any less of a woman? I don't think it's fair to say it does.

In my life I have a lot of kids, kids I would like to be there for: my nieces, my nephews, all of my friends' kids, my little cousins, some of my not-so-little cousins. There are a lot of kids out there who need someone to love them. And when I think about my favorite people growing up, many of them were not related to us or were, but not immediately. That thought brings me joy.

Plus. I think that knowing, watching and loving someone who struggles as you grow up makes you a kinder, more empathetic person who realizes that the world can be complicated and unexpected.

Though it is hard to think of a world where having a kid is not my choice, it's also nice to have a decision like this made for me. I guess.

Loneliness

Having cancer in my young adulthood has been a very lonely experience, and I imagine cancer is always pretty lonely. Despite the fact that it touches SO many people, you alone are experiencing it and you are seeing peers do things you always thought you'd be doing. For me, I go out and I can't really hear. I don't talk well so I can't really have a conversation. I also don't see great or process things as quickly as I used to. I'm in my own head a lot. And that's a pretty lonely place. I can be surrounded by people and feel like I'm totally by myself.

I have also isolated myself a lot, because I can't do what I used to be able to do and being alone is just so much easier. I don't think this is an answer to my problems, but it seems only natural. I don't want to be thought of as "the cancer patient", I want to be thought of as Katie, the athletic, pretty girl who is tough as nails.

This is kinda silly, because I don't think of any of my friends who have a disability as "representatives" of their illness or disability. I think of them as my friend, who I am there for and want to hang out with, but the story I'm telling myself is a different story. In my story, I am the monster, the burden, the downer.

I recently said to a good friend, "Wouldn't everything just be easier for Will if I weren't here?"

She looked at me and said, "Would it?"

I think she was partially talking about Will and partially talking about anyone who loves me. Like, sure they wouldn't have to deal with the inconveniences I cause, but they also wouldn't get any of the good things. This was very sweet of her to say, and it made me think about loneliness in a new way, in that we are all partially responsible for our own loneliness.

I choose to isolate myself and though there aren't many people who can know what I'm going through, there are plenty of people who can think about what their life would be if they felt like they'd lost everything.

Loneliness is a part of cancer—especially rare cancer—that no one prepared me for. At a time when I feel least like myself, I need to seek out others even more. There's definitely a mind-body connection, and I think feeling lonely and sad doesn't help anyone get better or fight for the life they have. I think we all need to feel like we matter—to someone other than our mothers. Think of it in animalistic, pure, survival terms: If we matter, we are more important to this earth. If we are more important to this earth, we are more likely to live. As animals we want to live, therefore mattering is inherent to our nature.

The Internet and television and movies (media)

I used to have a job. That meant eight hours/day I was out of the house, working hard. (Or hardly working!) Now I spend most of that time going to appointments, doing PT (less than I should), writing, and, of course, distracting myself with TV, movies, and the internet.

Now, the internet can be a really scary place for cancer patients, and I would definitely suggest that you DON'T Google your disease. First of all, the internet is full of worst-case scenarios, and second, the only time I googled my disease, my husband was out of town and I cried until I could not anymore, because the internet told me that I had very bad chances. Why I did this is anyone's guess, but I did.

The internet can also be an amazing place. There is so much out there to know and laugh at. You've seen my thoughts on social media, and social media is a huge part of the internet. I spend too much time on Facebook and Instagram, partially because I can connect with others from my couch, and partially because they're just plain entertaining.

Which is also why I watch a lot of TV and movies—I can feel like I get to go somewhere when I can't or I can get wrapped up in someone else's drama and think to myself, "Well, at least I don't have THAT going on."

Books are also great for this. There's nothing like a good book to take you somewhere you can't go: the past, the future, a place that doesn't really exist. I love to read—to laugh, to learn, and to escape—but my eyesight isn't great right now, which makes reading hard and slow (-er, than it already was! I've always been a slow reader!) That's a huge reason this book has taken me so long to write: Reading and typing are HARD. I guess that explains any typos....

TV and movies and books and the internet are great, but we also have to be responsible and active in our own lives. It's easy to be passive and go on the adventures of other people, but what adventures do we still have left? I don't want ALL of my stories to be someone else's stories or about CANCER. How boring.

So, write a book, go to the park, create your adventures where you can. Where you can't (because you physically can't or because the place you want to go does not exist), watch a show that you like.

Semantics

Since having cancer, I have not been a big fan of the nomenclature around the disease. People like to use words like "strong" and "warrior" and "survivor." What is the opposite of all of those things? Weak. Wimp. Loser.

I guess I'm sensitive. But words and language matter. They often impact how we feel about something, they can change over time, and they help us establish our whole identity. I remember a very common conversation the first week of college that was about whether you said "soda" or "pop"—the idea being that it could help determine where you were from, regionally.

Those who lose the "fight" against a disease are not weak or losers. And I know there is a collective "well duh" coming through, but I hear that terminology often enough that I think it bears discussion.

Cancer is evil and it takes things away from you. Telling you you're strong and a fighter and a warrior is really super NICE to hear when you're down in the trenches. But it's also a lot of pressure over something you can't control.

I don't think it's bad to say those things to someone when you believe them to be true and you want the person to fight and feel positive. But I just want everyone to be prepared for the idea that, sometimes, no matter how hard you fight, you don't win.

I'm not sure what the RIGHT nomenclature is, so I'm not very helpful here. But I guess the current language seems to leave out a lot of people who are very much in this disease.

Or maybe it doesn't. We don't consider soldiers who fight in lost wars "losers." We consider them heroes who fought for what they believed, despite the risks. We are definitely not winning the "War on Terror," but I do not blame that on any individual who has lost a leg or life fighting a war I would never join (largely because I don't believe in war, in general, but ESPECIALLY not this one, and because, let's face it, I'm a big, selfish wimp and war seems scary).

So I guess my point is that whenever you call a cancer patient a survivor, make sure they identify with it and that they understand that no matter what happens, they are a fighter and a winner.

Lance

Having cancer got me thinking a lot about Lance Armstrong, because he is the only famous person, I know of, to beat brain cancer.

How did he do it? I asked myself. So I did some reading. Turns out he had testicular cancer that had migrated to the brain, which is never good, but also, testicular cancer is considered one of the easiest cancers to treat, meaning the cancer in his brain had a very clear plan of action and was not a particularly aggressive form of cancer.

Also, Lance Armstrong was very rich, with a lot of prestige, and we cannot deny the importance of privilege when it comes to health issues. Access to insurance, medicine, care givers, etc. is all very expensive. Cancer is damn pricy. Which is why Universal Health Care needs to be a thing. But don't get me started on the flaws in our medical system....

Anyway, I think the real issue with Lance is that he stuck to his story of "not doping" for so long. 'Cause, I mean, what do you do if the whole game is rigged against you?? You play the game! I mean, if you're a really strong person, you don't play it and you call it out for what it is, but Lance probably has/had the heart of an athlete: He just wanted to win.

And it's possible that, like any human, at one point he lied, to keep his winning record. And then he had lied. And he felt he had to stick to it. And the longer he stuck to it, the truer it became for him.

It sucks that he let down so many people, especially those who were sick and turned to him as a sign of hope, but that footage of him, super skinny, in the hospital after treatment, on a bike, is real AND true. And also amazing. He probably felt like shit. I have taken some of the medicines he took and I can tell you, they do not make you feel like you want to ride a bike. They do make you feel like you want to lie on the couch and watch five seasons of Friday Night Lights (but, like, I never did that)....

Anyway, I have thoughts on Lance (shocker) and they're not all negative. I don't think he should have been stripped of all of his medals, but I'm not in charge of those kinds of decisions.

When you are famous, you get to be rich and have access to lots of things. But you are most definitely not allowed to be human.

Caring about the world when our world is small

Recently I bought a bamboo toothbrush and some shampoo and conditioner that don't come in plastic bottles. It reminded me of a story from when I was in college.

I remember being home and I needed to change my toothbrush. I was talking to my dad and saying I was freaking out a little about changing my toothbrush and how everyone has to change their toothbrush and how it was so much waste and it stressed me out and blah, blah, blah. I distinctly remember him saying to me "Katie, I don't think the world will be undone by toothbrushes." He just wanted his daughter to stop freaking out and change her damn toothbrush.

In a way, he's right. The world will be undone by the big things—corporations, cars, the MEDICAL INDUSTRY—not the little things, like toothbrushes. But he's also wrong. We, as little individuals, don't have much control when it comes to those big things, but we do have control in how we handle our own ish. If more people cut down on their plastic, in the tiniest ways, like where they get their toothbrush, it could have a really huge impact.

And it's always a choice. If brushing your teeth or using a certain shampoo that only comes in plastic containers is like the happiest thing ever or even if it's just kinda your "thing," then I think you keep on doing it. We do what we can and we mostly can't do everything. We live in a world and culture of consumerism. Escaping that is a huge effort and takes a lot of energy most of us just don't have. So we do what we can.

How does this relate to cancer? I guess it doesn't, really. Though, we are far less in control of our carbon footprint when we have to rely on others all of the time. But for all the things we can't agree on, we can probably agree that cancer sucks and that this world is objectively beautiful. And HEY GUESS WHAT??? WE ONLY GET ONE. They haven't found (to date) another planet that's like Earth with water and cool animals and an ecosystem like ours! So be nice to it. Humans are like the worst thing to happen to this planet. So do what you can.

I asked myself where I would be when my time to act came. Well I think it's here. And where am I? Stuck in my building. Sickly. Sitting around. While people march and rally and SHOW UP. All I can do is what I can do. That involves a lot of trying to make my life greener, to the extent that is possible for me. Sure, I could be doing a lot more, but I think that all or nothing attitude is what got us here in the first place.

I only have one planet, one life. I want to treat it like it's special and live it like I love it... the best I can, at any given moment

At this given moment, I am sick and I rely on my caretaker and my husband for ANYTHING I want to do, which includes joining marches, making money, and shopping for groceries. When my world is small, I can only do what's within my power to do. What is within your power? Are you doing what you CAN to save our planet?

I have become semi-obsessed with doing things "greenly" in the easiest way possible, which I sort of guess is not the point. Trying to take the easy way out is usually not green. But what else can I do?

Words

These are topics I have been thinking about a lot lately, and have taken on a different meaning since I've had cancer. They are also, let's be honest, just things I feel like opining on.

1. Gratitude

Will and I were recently in the Midwest in my childhood home. We went to surprise my mom but it was also kinda selfish: I wanted to be home for a little while.

I know that gratitude and being grateful are hot words right now and I think that is mostly a good thing: We should all focus on what we HAVE rather than focusing on what we don't have. Being home made me feel very, very grateful.

I have parents who love me and always made choices based on their kids' interests, not their own. I have a very loving and generous brother. My high school and childhood friends still give a shit about me (and travel far distances to see me). My college friends are very cool people. I grew up in a nice home located in a nice town with good, nay GREAT, schools. Most of all, I'm married to a wonderful human, who I barely deserve, and who makes it all possible to go back to Chicago in the first place. I could go on listing gratitudes until I'm blue in the face but I already feel like this is a long humblebrag anyway, so I'll stop.

One thing Will and I have started doing before we go to sleep is asking each other what we are grateful for THAT DAY. It doesn't have to be big or flashy, (like "family" or "friendship," though both of those things have definitely been said), but it should be something that made your day/life better.

I have said "Netflix."

It's a nice exercise. It helps to focus on the good when everything is so bad. I would suggest you try it, with a partner or on your own. It's a great way to combat anger and learn a little more about what's important to your partner and to you.

Also, sometimes, shitty is just shitty. If you don't feel like focusing on what you're grateful for, that's okay, too. Gratitude can be annoying when you're in the deep end. Like, when someone says, "Count your blessings...."

"Well okay, yeah, but that doesn't really help me right NOW."

For me, I feel really lucky to have what I've had in this life, but I'm not done with my lucky life. I know we all face hardships and that we all have to grow up. But it feels like the hits just keep on coming and I'm ready for some truly GOOD news.

Something my mother-in-law said that I have found really useful is that gratitude and suffering don't have to be opposing forces. You can be grateful for what you have, including the knowledge that there are others out there that have it "worse than you," while still acknowledging your own suffering.

I, like any normal human, can get into the comparison game: "Oh, you think that YOUR life is hard?" And, well, maybe for that person, it IS really hard. Suffering is suffering is suffering.

There are DEFINITELY whiners out there, and they should be held accountable, but just because someone else's pain is or has been bigger than yours, it doesn't mean your pain doesn't count.

Of course, pick who you complain to. (Like, I am not about to have sympathy for an adult who is scared of needles... actually, I probably will have sympathy—needles are scary as hell.) But I get so annoyed with the, "I have a cold... I know it's nothing like what you've gone through, but...."

I KNOW YOU KNOW THAT! DO YOU REALLY THINK I THOUGHT YOU WERE COMPARING YOUR COLD TO MY CANCER? Plus, colds SUCK and I ASKED you what was new!

I think the idea that gratitude and suffering can sit alongside one another has helped me play the "who has it worse?" game less. Yes, I am very grateful for the multitude of blessings my life has given (and still gives) me, but I have a rare brain cancer, and that fucking sucks.

2. Anger

I received a LOT of comments on a blog post I wrote about anger, which showed me two things: 1) This is an emotion that a lot of us feel and don't know what to do with; and, 2) If it ain't broke, don't fix it.

Anger

I've been thinking about this emotion a lot lately and have talked about it with two close friends. It is an emotion we don't like to talk about in this society because it is often ugly and violent, but it is also normal and natural. Yet, we are not taught how to deal with it. So we bottle it up and lash out. We hit and punch and cause destruction to others and our environment, because that's what we know. There HAS to be a healthy way to deal with anger. There are too many things in our world that are angering.

Cancer is one of them.

Trust me, I feel angry. And I haven't quite figured out what to do with it. A few weeks ago, I threw my phone on the ground (and really tested the case—no shattering, no external injuries). Then I threw a pillow and punched one until I was too tired to punch it anymore. So what lesson did I learn?

Well, 1) Boxers should be the least angry people on this planet; 2) My anger manifests itself very physically (duh, my brother is 6'6" and I spent my life as a competitive athlete); and 3) I am a lot angrier than I realized.

Of course I'm angry. I was young. I ate well. I worked out. I brushed my teeth (but I never flossed cause I'm lazy). Cancer has robbed me of many things, including youth. And so I feel pissed at the universe.

I recently read about this girl from Canada who is also named Katie (welcome to the 90's, ya'll) and was diagnosed with Stage IV breast cancer and, like, knew for a fact that she was going to die. She got a lot of attention because, despite this death sentence, she chose to focus on the positive.

Something about this story rubbed me the wrong way. Was I jealous of her? (Her fame? Her knowledge? Her ability to take a shituation and make something positive of it?)

I was definitely jealous of her fame and knowledge. I can't lie about that (or anything). I realized, though, that the emotion I was feeling was not actually directed toward her at all, it was directed at the COVERAGE of her. She was getting so much attention because, despite a shituation, she was still positive. I'm sure there is anger there—you don't get diagnosed with a terminal illness at age 31 without feeling a little bit angry about it, but she is not being celebrated for her realness. She is being celebrated for the opposite of that.

Don't get me wrong. I think she is amazing, and inspiring, all the good adjectives, but our society needs to figure out where to put anger. It's OK and normal. It only manifests itself in ugly because that's the only outlet we give it.

I was also thinking about anger in terms of sex and race, and how there are certain stereotypes around those things. Stereotypes are always damaging, but I think you can definitely see how much they just strip people of their humanity when it comes to an emotion we ALL feel, regardless of our skin tone or genitalia.

A black person acts angry and they play to the stereotype of the "angry black man/woman." A woman expresses anger, and "God, she's such a bitch." Would finding a healthy way to deal with this very common emotion mitigate the power of these stereotypes? I know it's all much deeper and more complicated than that, but could it help?

3. Fault

Fault is such a funny word because it has many definitions (one reason, among many, that English is such a difficult language).

One definition is like the fault in "fault line," as in geography, as in the fault line that slipped in California and caused that huge earthquake in the 90s... 80s? I don't even know.

There is supposed to be a giant earthquake coming in Seattle that will cause volcanoes to erupt and set off coastal tsunamis and ruin life as we know it. This is supposed to happen in… they don't know. Could be tomorrow, could be in another 100, 200, 500 years. The scientists really aren't sure.

I think shifting fault lines are just another way for the earth to say, "Get outta here, humans!! You are killing me and my only self-defense is to kill you!" I don't know, just a thought.

Then there's fault like someone's responsibility. I think about this a lot. When you get cancer, you really want someone to BLAME.

Is it God? No, I don't think so, because that would mean that if there WAS a God, she would be an evil one and I don't believe that God could be evil. Is it MY fault for using my phone as an alarm and eating a lot of Taco Bell in my teens? Well that certainly doesn't help anything.

I do think we are all responsible for making the world a more radioactive place. Sure, it's hard to know exactly whether there's actually more cancer with reporting and identification up from, say, 100 years ago, but I'm not sure it's deniable that our world is a more radioactive place. Everyone has a cellphone, often a "smart" phone (though mine can be pretty dumb sometimes) and the jury is still out on this one, but I'm fairly sure that all of the radiation that we emit all of the time makes our world a less safe place to be.

I'm not advocating for death to all smart phones—mine definitely means I spend a lot less time being lost, and it gives me something to do at 2 in the morning when I can't sleep. I'm only saying that you can't have your cake and eat it, too. (Another weird saying! What is the point of cake if not to be eaten??). If we want cell phones, GPS, microwaves, air travel, nuclear weapons*, etc., we will have to accept a world that is more radioactive. Therefore, there will be more cancer. Full stop.

And then there is fault as in problems. Like a person's faults, the things they should "work on."

Now, I'm not saying that we shouldn't all try to be better people, but I was also thinking about how my faults make me who I am. Without them, I'm not Katie. I'm not human. They not only give me something to work on, but they also make me ME.

I think that's something we all lose sight of. We try so hard to work out all our kinks that we lose sight of the fact that our kinks are part of who we are. If your fault is, like, murder or perpetuating racism, then who you are is probably a bad person. But even then, the anti-hero is all the rage. Ask HBO or any "Breaking Bad" fan.

Faults are also very subjective and situational. What some might view as foolhardy, others might view as brave. Shy can be viewed as timid or watchful. Being sick has made me wary of "capital T Truths." Fault doesn't seem to have one.

I guess I always was wary of the idea of True, but there is no capital T Truth about cancer other than that it sucks. We can all agree on that, no matter our "faults."

4. Grief

Grief is an interesting word when you are sick.

There is the grief of those around you who love you and wish you weren't feeling the pain that you are feeling.

I'm okay with accepting a world without nuclear weapons, just for the record.

There is the grief of doctors and nurses who want to help you, but don't really know how. They have mostly learned how to deal with this grief, but with GOOD doctors or nurses, it is palpable.

And then there's your own grief, about so many things from the big to the small.

Sure, I grieve in the traditional sense in that I think about and am scared of death. I grieve for my parents, and my husband, and my siblings who are taking this journey with me, and might have to watch their daughter, wife, sister die much earlier than they should have to, if at all. And I grieve for the life I could have known, one of playdates with my nieces and nephews, one of biking through the park on a warm afternoon, and one of getting up early for a yoga class I really like before work.

I was talking to my therapist about all of the things I was frustrated by: my eyesight, my balance, my speaking, the list goes on and on. Something she said to me was, "When you talk about all of this stuff the main emotion I'm getting is grief. You are grieving the loss of who you once were."

This helped me a lot, to frame it like that. Grief is pain over a LOSS. We feel grief when we feel like we have lost a crucial piece of our lives.

I often feel grief for other people, but maybe that is just sympathy or empathy. Like when my Grandmother died, I remember feeling sad FOR my mom, because she was sad and the idea of living in the world without a mom made (and still makes) me nauseous, but I didn't really KNOW my grandmother, so there wasn't REAL grief. (Plus, I was six, so I didn't really understand the idea of death.) Grief, TRUE grief, came later when I was old enough to recognize the loss—the loss of a grandparent, the loss of stories, and the loss of a life.

Seeing my losses as things to grieve helped me, because you can't live in a state of grief forever. You can be SAD about something always, but eventually, you have to let time work its magic.

VI. CONCLUSION

"Life is what happens when you are busy making other plans."

Medical Outcome

As of June, 2019, I have opted to stop chemotherapy.

It's not killing the cancer. It's not taking the physical deficiencies away. I do tolerate it fairly well but it makes me feel weird and it means more time in the hospital and less time feeling like myself while I do things that I actually LIKE to do. This includes physical therapy, acupuncture, travel, reading, and spending time with family and friends. Oh, and of course, binge-watching Netflix.

This decision could change and I'm open to that. But for now, I'd rather enjoy what I do have than pump my body with chemicals. I am waiting and hoping to get into a trial for medulloblastoma. It is run out of Seattle Children's Hospital and has lots of requirements. They are taking a break to rewrite it, based on what they have already learned, and once they do, they'll be back at it. That will hopefully be soon, but they have stopped responding to my husband's emails. Haha.

I have joined some Facebook groups that bring cancer patients together and I have found two women who also had medulloblastoma as young adults. Crazy! But it definitely helps me feel less alone.

When I started this book two years ago, I thought for sure I would be done with this whole episode by now. I thought I'd be looking back at a crazy time... but I am still fully in it.

I'm not an idiot. I do not think I will come out of this unscathed. But I have always been a medical anomaly, and I plan to continue down that path in beating this thing!

Facing the unknown future

None of us knows when our expiration date is. For all of us, the future is unknown. A lot of people have said things like, "Wow, you have been in Seattle a long time! You must like it!"

That's true. I think the Pacific Northwest, and Seattle, are great. But part of me is afraid to permanently leave the area where I first got cancer. It's silly, because cancer doesn't know or have geographical bounds. And there are cancer doctors basically everywhere. But one thing someone "jokingly" said once is that Seattle is the best place to get cancer.

I don't know if that's something to be proud of, but there ARE good docs and hospitals here. Not to mention plenty of research centers like the University of Washington, Fred Hutchinson, and the Seattle Cancer Care Alliance (SCCA). Truth is, I have no idea what's going to happen with me. As one doctor once said to me, "There is no protocol for treating you."

The future is a big unknown. But I suppose that's true for all of us. We hold on to the illusion of control, though. I don't really make big plans anymore, which I know is dumb, but it has been so hard to let go of the future I thought I had, the idea of doing that all over again is daunting. It's easier for me to make fewer plans for the long-term future.

I can't currently work and what does a career look like, anyway?! I felt like I was finally figuring out what kind of job I actually wanted to do, and then my job became worrying about my health and fighting cancer. This is something I think about a lot: What am I doing if I'm not fighting cancer?

I guess just living life, one day after the other, like we all do.

Death (practically and emotionally)

This is not something that people want to think about, but there IS a practical side to death (like what happens to your things and money and where you go when you pass and all of that unpleasant stuff).

One thing cancer forced me to do, that I really think everyone should do, is get my ducks in a row when it comes to dying.

I found out about a will in Washington State—how a living will is different from a last will and testament (actually, I still don't totally understand this), and I had to make decisions about what would happen if I die.

Luckily, in my senior year of college I had the privilege of taking a religious studies class called "Meanings of Death," with Royal Rhodes. The main premise of the class, as I understood it, was that death is a very human thing and no matter your religious beliefs, your religion probably deals with death. One religion may do it differently than another, but we all think about it and we all experience it, so we might as well talk about it and come to terms with it before it happens.

Anyway, this class was very emotional and philosophical, but it also forced me to think about some of the practicalities surrounding death, ESPECIALLY since I didn't and don't have a religion with clear rules on how to handle my passing. It's kinda up to me.

Like, did you know that federal law prohibits states from requiring a coffin at all, and that it's the coffin INDUSTRY (Big Coffin?) that makes people think they have to pay big bucks for a fancy box to be buried in?

You can literally be buried in a shroud. And depending on the state and zoning laws and all that, you can be buried ANYWHERE. This fascinated and still fascinates me.

Cancer has forced me to face these practicalities at a young age. Basically I learned that making a will doesn't mean you have to turn anything in, or have anything notarized, or any of that business. I mean, you should see what your state rules are, but where I live, you just have to have things written down. Then you should probably share that document with someone you trust. For me, it is my husband. I talked to a social worker and looked up state laws, and then I made a Google Doc* that I shared with Will that included instructions on what to do with my assets (there are very few), what to do if there are machines involved, and what I want at my memorial.

I know that memorials are largely for the living, or at least I think they are. But I have some small requirements of a memorial for me.

Cancer or not, my larger point is that everyone should do this. I hope everyone lives a long life where something like this isn't needed at a young age, but the reality is that none of us knows when we'll die. The last thing I want to do to already-grieving family is give them more hard decisions to make.

I remember reading once, "I never thought much about life BEFORE I existed, why would it be any different after?"

I like this thought but I also wonder if it's different once you've actually experienced life—like when you learn the meaning of a word and you start seeing that word everywhere? Don't you miss people? Don't you miss certain smells and feelings? I won' pretend to know, but I do wonder.

I am not getting money from Google to promote their document service, though I kinda wish I was....

The idea of souls is lovely, and I believe in it, but is it selfish? Is it just another way for humans to ascribe meaning to the meaningless? Certain things do seem fated. I, and many others, have had a supernatural experience, and I have met people who DEFINITELY seem like "old souls," wise beyond their years.

I am still very afraid of death. Even if it's "an end to suffering" it's also an end to the world as we know it, and though I know that things will go on and everyone will be fine, non-existence is a hard thing to wrap my mind around. It reminds me a lot of when I went to go visit a favorite high school teacher after my freshman year of college. I knew on some level that everything just keeps going, but seeing all of the old familiar hallways, and seeing my old favorite teachers surrounded by new students... it was just unsettling.

We all think about death and we all die. Disease makes you think about it earlier than you might have to otherwise. I've thought a lot about death and what it would mean if I did not exist, and it makes me sad for two reasons: 1) the hurt it would cause the people I love; and, 2) there are still so many things I want to do. Oh, and 3) life is really painful but it's also really beautiful. I am still amazed at the number of times the beauty of this Earth takes my breath away.

The idea of not having any breath to take away makes me feel sad.

Why?

"I find that the harder I work, the more luck I seem to have."
--Thomas Jefferson

So, why did I write this book? Well, for many reasons.

One, I've always liked to write to process hard things. Two, reading gives us knowledge, power, escape, and perspective; that's why I've always considered books awesome. And, three, I'm a self-important jerk who thinks my experiences are important to capture!

No. I really wrote this book because throughout many of these last months and years I've felt very alone and I don't want other people to have to feel alone in the same way. Young adults go through illness too, and however you go through it is how you go through it! We all often wish things were different, but they're not.

I think, ill or healthy, we draw a lot of lines in our lives: We ARE a certain way. We BELIEVE in certain things. We DO whatever for a living. We can HANDLE x but definitely not y....

Lines can be helpful—we draw them for reasons—but we have to learn where they are helpful and where they are just constraining. I think you learn how to dance many lines when you are ill. Sometimes your dance is a lot more rhythmic than at others.

One time, I said to a friend, "Don't you ever just feel like it's too late [to try something new]?" And, without skipping a beat, she says, "No." For her, the lines are flexible and ever-changing, as I think they need to be.

I expected my life to go one way and then it didn't. Should I try to keep pushing that boulder up the hill or should I stop and go to a different hill?

The more things that cancer takes away from me, the more I realize that trying to change that which we cannot is like hitting our heads against the wall. It's an entirely Sisyphean task.

I don't say this like I am giving up; it would be AMAZING if everything went back to the way it was. But I think the more I keep trying that, the more I fail and the less I am acknowledging what it DOES take to get through this disease, or other illness... or life:

Grace, tenacity, humility... and some luck, here and there.

AFTERTHOUGHT:
TRITE BULLSHIT I WANTED TO INCLUDE BUT COULDN'T FIND THE RIGHT SPOT FOR

"Agree to disagree."

"People in glass houses shouldn't throw stones."

"You miss 100% of the shots you don't take."

"Where there's a will, there's a way."

"If you want to make God laugh, show him your plans."

"We'll cross that bridge when we come to it."

"Anything worth doing isn't easy."

"The only thing consistent in life is change."

"What doesn't kill us only makes us stronger."

"Tough times require tougher people."

Katie Weber was born Kathleen Willis Weber in Arlington Heights, Illinois, just outside Chicago. She is technically a "millennial," she admits, but can clearly remember the days before cell phones were "a thing." She feels this is an important distinction.

Tall and athletic, she was an avid high school basketball and soccer player. Before "all of this cancer crap," she notes, she loved to do yoga, ride her bike, walk everywhere, and take the bus while listening to podcasts. She chronicles her thoughts about life and the lemons she's been handed on her blog, *"You never really know a person until you...climb into his skin and walk around in it."* (https://cancerthoughtsandmore.wordpress.com.)

She is happily married to a "wonderful guy" she met at Kenyon College in Ohio. They live in Seattle.

Made in the USA
Middletown, DE
04 May 2020

92643181R00070